DISCOVER YOUR VOICE
HOW TO DEVELOP HEALTHY VOICE HABITS

DISCOVER YOUR VOICE
HOW TO DEVELOP HEALTHY VOICE HABITS

■

OREN L. BROWN

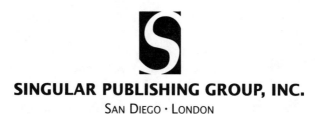

SINGULAR PUBLISHING GROUP, INC.
SAN DIEGO · LONDON

Singular Publishing Group, Inc.
401 West A Street
San Diego, California 92101-7904

19 Compton Terrace
London, N1 2UN, UK

Typeset in 10/12 Bookman by So Cal Graphics
Printed in the United States of America by McNaughton & Gunn

Library of Congress Cataloging-in-Publication Data
Brown, Oren.
    Discover your voice : how to develop healthy voice habits / by
Oren L. Brown.
        p.   cm.
    Includes bibliographical references and index.
    ISBN 1-56593-704-X
    1. Voice—Care and hygiene.   2. Singing—Instruction and study.
  I. Title.
MT821.B86 1996
783'.04—dc20   96–194
                                                                  CIP
                                                                   MN

CONTENTS

■

Foreword

■

The name "Oren Brown" has been prominent in the field of voice for half a century. His expertise as a singing teacher has been recognized around the world. However, in addition to a well-deserved reputation as a fine singing teacher, Oren Brown is recognized as a pioneer in the evolution of voice care as a medical subspeciality. He was one of the first singing teachers to work regularly in a medical setting, collaborating with an otolaryngologist long before interdisciplinary teams were popular. He recognized the value of enhancing traditional approaches to voice training, utilizing scientific concepts and methodology. Through seminars in many countries, extensive private teaching, and years on the faculty of prestigious institutions such as the Juilliard School of Music, he helped educate generations of teachers and performers to be receptive to scientific ideas, research, and creative thought about pedagogical approaches. His efforts were exceedingly effective in helping to overcome the widespread resistance among teachers and singers to close scrutiny, scientific analysis, and intellectual challenge. The foundations he laid have been invaluable not only in facilitating the evolution of voice into an interdisciplinary medical subspecialty, but also in allowing voice pedagogy to evolve into a more sophisticated and scientific discipline.

Discover Your Voice: How to Develop Healthy Voice Habits synthesizes Brown's personal practices, thoughts, and techniques. This book distills decades of practical experience. Because of Mr. Brown's contributions and prominence, this work is of substantial historical interest. In addition, it provides a great deal of information from the perspective of a scientifically oriented singing teacher that is practical and invaluable to singers and their teachers. He includes a considerable amount of factual information and wonderful insights into the importance of scientific knowledge in the voice studio. This book should be a valuable addition to the library of any singing teacher, singer, or other professional interested in the singing voice.

Robert T. Sataloff, M.D., D.M.A.

Preface

■

This book fulfills a promise I've made to my students for many years to expand a 19-page syllabus outlining the basic principles of healthy voice use. "It's our bible," a teacher in Wisconsin wrote recently. "We're waiting for the book."

Here it is . . . finally.

The story starts in 1952 with Dr. Theo Walsh—a man with imagination, courage, and a problem. Head of the Department of Otolaryngology at Washington University School of Medicine in St. Louis, Missouri, Dr. Walsh realized that a number of patients with functional voice disorders did not respond to treatment offered by surgeons, psychiatrists, and other members of the staff. He decided to try an experiment, that is, to engage someone who knew voices from another point of view. He offered the job to me, but I hesitated. Although I had been teaching singing for almost 20 years in Boston and St. Louis, "voice therapy" as we know it today was still an unchartered science.[1] To reassure me, Dr. Walsh said that doctors were trained to use their eyes, but that I had been trained to use my ears; and ears were needed, he thought, to understand many vocal problems. It was a challenge. I agreed to divide my time between their clinic at Barnes Hospital and my private voice studio, and the arrangement continued for 16 years.

Dr. Walsh was enthusiastic and generous. He gave me a white coat, showed me how to use the laryngeal mirror and invited me to attend weekly staff meetings. My youngest patients were 4 and 5 years old; the oldest, over 80. There were men and women from many walks of life, in various stages of difficulty. In a clinic where time and money were always in short supply, results were essential. Literature on voice disorders was sparse at that time. Consequently, I relied on intuition to supplement my

---

[1]It wasn't until 1964 that I attended a 5-day course on "Voice Disorders of Children," given at Central Missouri State College, with enrollment limited to 30. To my knowledge, this course was the first of its kind presented in the United States.

experience as a musician and teacher to develop methods that would change the life-long habits of these troubled people.

Working closely with doctors who had referred their patients to me, I was happy to find that a gratifying percentage were rehabilitated by exercises and other forms of treatment. Because the disorders were diverse, the "cures" also were diverse.

My work at the Barnes Hospital clinic was exciting and extremely rewarding. I saw lawyers, ministers, and salesmen return to their jobs after visits of only a few weeks. The biggest thrill for me was to see a singer whose promising career had been stopped short by a polyp recover without surgery, audition for a new role, and get it! During my years in Dr. Walsh's department, over 2,000 patients reinforced my beliefs in the basic principles and techniques of healthy phonation.

In my private studio, my teaching was given a scientific foundation. I developed an altered pair of ears—far more sensitive than the ears Dr. Walsh originally employed. I listened for musicianship first, that is, the artist's attempt to express the composer's and his or her own thoughts and feelings. But because of my work at the clinic at the same time, I was on the alert for the initial signs of a sound which, if unchecked, would produce problems similar to those of patients streaming into the clinic. The imperative for me was—and still is—to help each and every artist develop habits that free them to achieve their goals.

Acknowledgments

■

I am greatly indebted to Arthur Wilson, with whom I studied singing for ten years in Boston. Much of what I was able to contribute at Barnes Hospital came from Mr. Wilson. I also owe much to David Blair McClosky, who introduced me to Dr. Walsh.

My gratitude for information, inspiration, and encouragement extends to all of the doctors on the staff at Washington University School of Medicine and the faculty of the Central Institute for the Deaf in the years 1952–1968. Thanks are due to the late Friedrich Brodnitz, MD., Paul Moses, MD., Hans von Leden, MD., Henry Rubin, MD., and Paul Moore, Ph.D., all of whom were most generous in sharing their knowledge of the vocal function. Along with all serious students of voice science, I take a deep bow to William Vennard, D.Mus., whom I am honored to have known as a friend.

Meetings of the American Academy of Otolaryngology were of priceless educational value. (I was privileged to give voice therapy courses at Academy meetings held in 1955 and 1956.) In 1957, the many voice scientists, speech-language pathologists, and doctors I met in Chicago at the International Voice Conference gave me a global perspective on the scientific investigations underway from that period on.

My thanks to the National Association of Teachers of Singing for that first summer workshop held at Indiana University in 1949, for inviting me to serve on its research committee and, for six years, as chairman of its Committee on Vocal Education.

Thank you, Sandra Kungle, D.Mus., for transcribing recordings of the lectures at my first voice seminar in Amherst, Massachusetts, in 1972. The transcripts were the first step toward creating this book. And thanks to Harry Hollein, Ph.D., for his critical examination of my syllabus, 1981, the second step towards this book.

For their editing of special chapters, I thank my son, Benjamin L. Brown, Ph.D., Physical Facts; Janet Graves-Wright, MM., MS., CCC., Voice Problems and Therapy; Richard Westenberg, DFA,

Choral Singing; Alix B. Williamson, Requirements for a Professional Career. I owe special thanks to Scott Kessler, MD, for his illustrations in this book. For helping me get started on the right track in the opening chapters, I thank David Brewer, MD; and for her appraisal of the first half of the manuscript, Linda Carroll, MS., CCC-SLP.

I especially thank the late Wilbur James Gould, MD, Ira Sanders, MD, and Ingo Titze, Ph.D., for their reading of the entire manuscript with special attention to the scientific material in Chapters XV through XVIII. I also thank the singing teachers David and Nancy Adams, Shirley Meier, and Janette Ogg, D.Mus., plus her two students in Vocal Pedagogy, Wendy DeLeo and Kimberly Pace, who also examined the entire manuscript.

For countless hours in editing, my sincere gratitude to Sarah Heartt, for 15 years a professional writer and editor; and to James Jones, longtime friend and student, for his many hours spent typing the manuscript.

Others are acknowledged at appropriate places in the text. My apologies to any whom I may have overlooked.

Finally, I express my undying gratitude to my late wife Juliska, without whose tireless support over many years this book might never have been written.

Introduction

■

Learning to sing is a process of discovering what your voice can do for you. It isn't so much a matter of *making sounds* as it is a matter of learning how to *let sounds happen.* Through experimentation, you become aware of what is taking place. By a process of selection, you reinforce what is easy through repetition.

I sometimes say that the three letters, L E T, spell the biggest word in learning how to use your voice. Merriam-Webster's *New Collegiate Dictionary* (1981) gives two meanings that support my emphasis: 1. to give opportunity to whether by positive action or by failure to prevent; 2. to free from or as if from confinement: RELEASE (She~out a scream). Everything that you were born with as a vocalist is still available. You only need a simple understanding of how your voice functions, an awareness of what is happening, and a will to put it to use.

This book provides information on what you have to work with, how you can exercise to develop your voice, and why the approach is healthy. The ideas are based on clinical and scientific evidence. Proof of their value has been demonstrated in seminars I have held each summer in Amherst, Massachusetts (1972–1985) and in Scandinavia since 1980. Countless teachers who have attended these meetings have written telling how much the ideas conveyed have benefitted their students.

If there were ever a study that could produce either healthy or harmful results, it is the study of singing. I have written this book so that others can avoid the delays and setbacks I experienced in my early years as a singer.

In the opening chapter, you will learn what your voice is and how you can discover it for yourself. The next chapter explains why an activity as simple as singing is so difficult and gives you relaxation and breathing exercises in Chapters II and III to make it easier.

In the following chapters, the exercises are so simple in the early stages that students often feel they are not doing enough. These exercises discussed in each chapter are illustrated with a score in the appendix and accompanied on compact disk. When students discover a new quality in their voices, they often exclaim that they don't know how they did it. I say to them, "Good! Do it again. Only this time, see if you can become aware of what is happening." Understanding the source of your sound and why it works the way it does can put to rest all thought of trying to "make" a sound.

Learning to integrate the wide vocal range given to you by nature has been called the ultimate in vocal technique by Dr. Henry Rubin. This book gives you exercises to bring about this integration and explains how the exercises help you.

As your voice develops, you will become eager to explore what can be done with it. Forming words and conveying their meaning brings you into a whole new world. You will find that your voice responds to your mental image. What and how you think become increasingly important as you develop vocal technique. The means by which you can progress are presented in a sequence of unfolding patterns which have no limits beyond the artist in each of you.

Many skills besides healthy voice use are needed for a successful career. "What ever happened to Mary . . . Tom . . . Betty . . . ?" my students ask me. So often a promising young artist fades into oblivion. For this reason, Chapter XIII is devoted to stimulating your thinking beyond the voice itself.

Chapter XIV, dedicated to choral singing, looks at what happens when people sing together, and the strengths and insights one can gain in a choral situation.

For the kind of student and teacher who want to have scientific explanation, I have written brief chapters on Physics (XV), Anatomy and Physiology (XVI), Neurology and the Brain (XVII), Hearing (XVIII), and Psychology (XIX), as these apply to singing. These chapters are especially significant for anyone who seeks a deeper understanding of the information given in the chapter on Voice Problems and Therapy (XX).

The closing chapter (XXI) is directed to the voice teacher—and every singer is his or her own teacher. The ideas presented are intended to stimulate your observation, your awareness of what teachers need to keep in mind. No matter how hard we try, we can never get inside a student's body or brain. Yet, the better we empathize, the better we can lead a student to an understanding of his or her own voice.

Have fun!

I

■

PRIMAL SOUND

When I asked Celia how she felt when she suddenly let go and released a glorious flood of tone, she exclaimed, "I feel naked! IT FEELS OUT OF CONTROL!" Celia had experienced her primal sound.

Have you ever had an experience like that? Do you know what I am talking about? Do you know what kind of sound you make when you laugh or cry or when you are startled, hurt, or disappointed?

You were given a voice just as you were given a face, arms, and legs. That voice is yours and yours alone, just as your face and body are yours and yours alone. The reason your voice seems mysterious is because you can't see it or put your hands on it. It's just there. This chapter is devoted to helping you understand your primal sound.

Primal sounds are involuntary. They are the sounds you were born with. In Beijing, Basel, or Boston, a baby's cry at birth is his primal sound. In 1963, Peter F. Oswald made a phonetic analysis of the baby cry. He labeled the initial sound as a schwa [ə], (*uh* as in *a*bout), which linked the cry to a baby's first word, "mama" [məmə]. "Mama" is the first word spoken by babies throughout the world. In Korea, the word is "ama," with the vowel preceding the consonant.

Think of the primal sounds of other animals. A dog barks, a horse neighs, a cat meows. When I ask an audience what the human sound is, they often answer, "talking." But speech is a man-made invention. By changing the shape of your mouth, tongue, lips,

1

and throat, the primal sound that originates in your larynx becomes molded into what we call vowels and consonants. Different combinations of these sounds create language or "talking."

Malcolm H. Hast (1983) writes that "the needs of an animal probably determine its phonatory activity—the repertoire of functions being recognition, mating, social organization, territoriality, etc." (p. 6). Darwin said that "sounds of a musical nature were first developed as a means of courtship and were associated with man's strongest emotions: love, rivalry and triumph" (1955, p. 87).

Outbursts of anger or alarm are universal in the animal kingdom. We humans, like all animals, create sound to express our various states and needs. These sounds are involuntary; they spring from our emotions. The nerve center for the emotions lies in the "lower brain." There is a direct connection from this area of the brain to the cortex or "upper brain"—the part with which we think.

FUNCTIONS OF THE LARYNX

Chevalier Jackson and his son Jackson Jr. (1937) identified nine different functions of the larynx. One of these was called a *reflexive sound*, which produces emotional expression, another, the *voluntary production of sound* corresponding to the sounds that come from the lower (emotional) and upper (thinking) brain. Primal sound, then, is the reflexive sound which produces emotional expression. It is the sound you make without thinking when, for example, you are amused or startled or enraged.

The word *primal* has the connotation of being first, new, initial, uncopied, unique, basic, fundamental, original. That is why I chose it.

Every person has a throat as distinct and individual as his or her face. (Think of it: Your voice is as unique as your face.) As an illustration of how distinct each throat is, I will describe an incident in the clinic at Barnes Hospital many years ago. I asked the supervising doctor to check a patient he had referred to me for voice therapy a month earlier. The doctor looked at the patient's face and said he had never seen the man before.

"But, Doctor," I exclaimed, "your referral is recorded here in the chart."

"That must be someone else's handwriting," he replied. "But, I'll take a look if you want me to." Whereupon he adjusted his head mirror and proceeded to examine the patient's throat. "Oh, yes!" he exclaimed. "Now I remember." The doctor recalled details of the patient's throat but didn't recognize the patient's face!

If everyone has a throat as distinct as one's face, it is logical to assume that one will have a voice that is distinctly one's own. Perhaps you have had the experience of answering the telephone and hearing the voice of a friend whom you have not seen for many years, yet you immediately recognize his voice.

Each individual has his or her own "voice print"—as distinctive as one's fingerprint. This should give you a sense of how very special you are—one of a kind—and explain why it is so important that you develop an awareness of what your voice feels and sounds like without imitating any other voice.

FREE YOUR VOICE

Your involuntary sounds are just as characteristic of you as the involuntary sounds of other animals are of them. The question is, how much can you trust the sounds you make when you are not thinking? Children rarely stop to wonder why they are able to cry or laugh or talk. Nor do they stop to think *how* they do it. They just let it out. It is difficult to trust what will happen if you let your primal sounds out, but that is exactly what we *must do*.

You have this ability! Do you recognize it? Do you use it when you sing? Do you know how to keep it running through your repertoire? Perhaps you fear you will look foolish if you show your inner feelings. Do you perceive it as a sign of weakness?

As a student of voice, you need to rediscover what it is to become as a little child, free from all inhibitions. You must reestablish contact with your instinctive being so that you can strip away the habits that stand in the way of learning how your voice behaves naturally. In this context, the essence of healthy voice production is the primal sound.

You may say that this is all very well, but you are no longer a child. That is just the point. You must rediscover yourself. To quote from Robert Masters (1975): "In the present normal course of human development, even by the end of the third year of life, coordination has become impaired in most persons" (p. 30).

Almost from birth, children are conditioned by their surroundings. While there is no danger in being your true, natural self, imitation has its costs. I remember asking a group of medical interns to count from one to five, in order to sample their speaking voices. When each had finished, I asked one of them if his voice got tired after speaking for 15 or 20 minutes. "I don't know why you pick on me," he replied. "Everyone says I sound exactly like my father and grandfather." The next day his throat was examined by the head of the Department of Otolaryngology and the day after that he was admitted for removal of vocal polyps.

This story is unusual, yet it shows that habits acquired in youth can be detrimental later in life. Many people whom I had as patients had histories of vocal malfunction going back to infancy. From birth, the sounds we make are conditioned by our surroundings. Imitation can be a blessing or a curse. As children, how can we differentiate good voice use from the unnatural strains of imitation? Add to this that recorded music (also a Broadway show) is altered by sound technicians, and it is no wonder that we reach adulthood having lost touch with our primal sound.

What can you trust? Your primal sound! Get to know it. Find out who *you* are. Explore! Experiment! Release old habits to make way for the new.

When I hear great singing, it is as though I were listening to a marvelous animal. I believe this is why audiences are so deeply moved by great singing. At a subconscious level, empathy takes place when a singer shares his or her primal sound.

I used to adore Claudia Muzio (1889–1936), whom I heard in Boston in my youth. Many years later I met a man who had been a friend of hers. He told me that she once confessed, "I don't know how I do it." I'm sure this is true of a great many singers born with talent and fortunate to have good guidance as they grow and mature. A much larger percentage could succeed if they knew how to transfer primal sound into trained, conditioned responses.

RELATIONSHIP BETWEEN THINKING AND VOCALIZING

Because we make sounds so naturally, most people do not realize that the vocal folds come together just by thought. In recent years an instrument called the flexible fiberscope has been used to examine the larynx. With this instrument you can see your own vocal folds on a video screen. A cough, laugh, or cry can be easily demonstrated. From an open position of ordinary breathing, the folds will jump together to produce a variety of sounds, responding to voluntary or involuntary stimuli.

Using the flexible fiberscope and video screen, one of my students experimented with her voice during a series of tests conducted by the late Van L. Lawrence of Houston, Texas. This student wrote a list of different tasks to see what would happen as she watched the movements of her vocal folds on the screen. On finishing her list, she turned to me for suggestions. I sounded a note on a pitch pipe and asked her to *think* it, but make no sound. Pop! The vocal folds came into position, ready to make a sound. I asked her to think of a tone an octave higher and the folds took on a different formation. She exclaimed, "I've often heard you say that the vocal folds will adjust automatically just by thinking—and there's the proof!"

All the vocal qualities you were born with are there, ready to use, if you can only find the key to unlock them. They are a function of the autonomic nervous system, which has been conditioned to respond to the efferent nervous system.

Some of the great singers of the past must have sensed this relationship between thinking and vocalizing. Nellie Melba (1922), said "Simply think the note and allow it to come" (p. 26). I'm sure that Melba and others did not know *why* this worked, but their approach produced some marvelous results. With what we know today, it is our responsibility to guide students so that they, too, can simply "think the note and allow it to come out."

WORKING WITH YOUR EMOTIONS

Where can we find examples of well-conditioned primal sound? Caruso had it. Chaliapin had it. So did Ponselle, and Callas, and Flagstad. They had it because they were able to inject emotional experiences from their own lives into the words and music they sang. If lacking direct experience, these performers had the imagination to project themselves into the music in a way that made the listener feel as though the performer were living the text.

Caballe, Domingo, Horne, and Pavarotti "grab our gut." Their singing brings tears to our eyes or puts us on the edge of our seats in suspense. We empathetically groan, moan, laugh, cringe, lament, rejoice, or become exhausted with despair. To be sure, the feelings have to be in the music, but without a singer who can express them, we are cheated of the full experience we might otherwise enjoy.

"That's all very well," you say, "but what am I supposed to do?"

FINDING YOUR PRIMAL SOUND

Nothing takes the place of trying sounds for yourself. As a starter, just say "Huh!" [hə], as if reacting in surprise to an astonishing statement. Now try "Uh huh" [əhə], as in an expression of agreement. Next, try "Huh-huh" [həhə], as in a laugh. Don't worry if you feel silly doing this. Everyone does at first. The sound people make when they don't know what they want to say is a prolonged "uh" [əh]. Try this sound. Now, extend this into a long sigh, "Huh" [həh] (Example #1; see vocal exercises in appendix and on compact disc).

Next, prolong the "Huh" and let the sound slide up and down (Example #2). You will notice that as the tone goes up it seems to get lighter or brighter and, by contrast, seems heavier or darker in the lower range. This is the way nature intended. For now, keep everything as simple as possible. Realize that what seem to be changes in quality between high and low are natural responses.

Here is something else to try. Take a comfortably full breath and start a kind of crying or whining sound, prolonging it until you are out of breath, and letting it slide around, up and down. (Huh—) (Example #3). This can go for a long time.

If you have succeeded in the above, say "Huh" [həh] in an extended downward sigh. Repeat, starting a bit higher, then lower (Example #4). Now, see if you can produce a light laugh and prolong the last sound (Example #5).

You are making a neural bridge between the lower brain that releases emotional expression and the upper part that thinks (the cortex). You have started to bring a natural function into a willed action. This link to your primal source is most desirable. Both speech and song come out of this kind of phonation. It is like the trunk of a tree, with speech being a branch in one direction and song a branch in another. The better you are able to discover your primal sound, the easier it will be to trust, train, and employ that sound in your art.

We practice in order to sensitize responses by thinking and singing definite pitches a bit at a time over many years. A young child will not be as accurate as a young adult, and a young adult will not be as efficient as a highly trained singer. Moreover, each singer must proceed at his or her own pace. Each starts with a different combination of assets and liabilities. This is what makes learning and teaching such a challenge. If, however, each step is mastered, in due time, you will find yourself gradually replacing negative patterns with positive patterns. Can you imagine how wonderful it would be if you only practiced sounds that were good for you?

SUMMARY

Learning to sing is like learning to juggle. You begin with just one object and in time a second and a third can be added. It takes an incredible amount of patience, but to hurry the process would merely defeat the outcome. It is in trying to do too much too soon that many a fine natural talent has been ruined.

First and foremost, find your primal sound. It doesn't matter whether you are just beginning or have been singing for years. If you locate your primal sound, you are on your way to realizing your full potential as an artist. If you don't, your growth will be stunted.

Do you think you speak with this sound? Do you speak with it all the time or just sometimes? Many people have gotten into habits of speech that have led them away from their primal sound. You must develop a healthy speaking voice to develop a healthy singing voice.

Beverly Sills once said that when she was a girl her father kept telling her to lower her voice. She thought he meant a lower pitch rather than a softer sound, so she developed a low speaking range compared to the average lyric-coloratura soprano.

I knew a young woman who talked and sang with a light, breathy quality. She sang for a panel of voice teachers to find out what could be done to correct this condition, but nothing they tried seemed to work. Finally, a teacher in the audience requested permission to ask her a question. "What do you do for a living?" he asked. "I work in a library," she almost whispered. Through acquiring the habit of speaking softly in the library, she had completely lost touch with her primal sound.

Many more stories could be told to illustrate how people acquire habits that interfere with their use of a free, natural voice. There is an extended discussion of this in Chapter XX, entitled Voice Problems and Therapy.

With this knowledge as a foundation, you are ready to take the next step in learning how to *let* your voice *happen*. This is an ideal to strive for; it lies at the root of great vocal performance. It may take a lifetime of study. Often, the greatest accomplishments have very simple truths behind them. This is why primal sound is so important. We are tapping a resource that is basic to all mammals' nature.

- Primal sound is the key for the artist in you to communicate as a singer.
- Primal sound is the key for the thinker in you to reach your audience as a speaker.
- Primal sound is essential for your vocal health as a singer or speaker.

Think! Let! Pray! Trust!

REFERENCES

Darwin, C. (1955). *The expression of the emotions in man and animals*, (p. 87). New York: New York Philosophical Library (Original work published 1896).

Hast, M.H. (1983). *Vocal fold physiology*, (p. 6). Denver, Co: Denver Center of the Performing Arts.

Jackson, C., & Jackson, C.L., Jr. (1937). *The larynx and its diseases*. Philadelphia: Saunders.

Masters, R. (1975, February 22). *Saturday Review*, (p. 30).

Melba, N. (1922). *The Melba method*, (p. 26) (article). London: Chapell.

Ostwald, P.F. (1963). *Soundmaking*, Springfield, Il: Charles C. Thomas.

II

■

RELEASE

I use the term *release* to describe the attitude needed to let your voice convey its full potential. Press a light switch and the light goes on. An Olympic diver stands ready to perform, then he "presses a button" and goes through the movements he has programmed through months or years of training, and "plip!"—enters the water with hardly a splash.

What could you do to improve your potential? My advice is to keep out of the way. Allow all possible freedom to carry out the conditioned response.

LEARNING TO RELAX YOUR MUSCLES

You sing with your whole body. Many of your body functions are cared for by your involuntary nervous system, the animal in each of you. Primal sound is an automatic response, which you can improve by learning to keep out of its way. The essence of vocal technique is to perform with the greatest freedom and the least effort.

Your larynx is suspended freely in your throat. Good vocal production depends on keeping the surrounding muscles as free from strain as possible. Any undue pull from the outside will throw the inner adjustments out of balance. This is why lifting is not a good exercise for singers. Muscles in the neck and shoulders become tense.

One of the nine functions of the vocal folds is called *fixative*. In lifting, or in placing any similar strain on the body, the vocal folds are set firmly in a closed position to stabilize the breath pressure in the lungs. This gives the larger body muscles a steady base for physical activity. Athletes use the fixative position for feats of strength. For making sound, the opposite is needed—freedom of movement in the larynx.

Most interfering tensions are acquired. This means you need to get back to your native self—to rediscover what will happen if you *let* your larynx hang free.

Muscular stress in the larynx is called *hyperfunction*. This is the root of most vocal problems. There are a number of ways to bring about release. Some can be passive, such as through meditation, while others involve a series of exercises.

Muscles are stimulated for action through the nervous system. Nerves travel from the brain down through the neck and spine to the various parts of the body. In singing and speaking, therefore, it is very important to have the entire spinal column (including the neck) as free from stress as possible.

Because of the sympathetic nervous system, an injury to one part of the body can be reflected in other parts of the body. According to *Gray's Anatomy*, "the sympathetic system mobilizes the energy for sudden activity such as that in rage or flight" (Lea & Febiger, 1954, p. 1087). If you accidentally pounded your fingers with a hammer, you would probably say, "Ouch!" and make all manner of grimaces. A pain in one part of the body can cause tension in the throat. Therefore, attention should be given to any bodily discomfort to help eliminate potentially unfavorable reactions in the phonating system.

We are all subjected to conditioning influences when we are young. While many are good, others are not part of our natural body state. Our nervous system is complicated; a main nerve often has several branches. For example, the vagus nerve, the one that controls your vocal folds, has branches that go to your lungs and stomach. Your tongue and jaw are served by a single nerve stem. Because the base of your tongue is attached to the hyoid bone from which your larynx is suspended, a tense jaw can affect the free adjustment of your vocal folds. (See Chapter XVII on Neurology and the Brain.)

Become aware of interfering tensions and find a way to free them. The exercises in this chapter will help you reestablish an uninhibited release of energy.

WORKING WITH YOUR SPEAKING VOICE

By the time you decide to study voice, you are probably already using habits that are not needed—habits you acquired unconsciously. This can apply to both speaking and singing. Because most of us talk more than we sing, speaking habits also need attention.

A young man with a very rough speaking voice came to study singing with me. When I told him that we needed to give attention to his speaking voice before we started on his singing, he said, "Everyone always told me that singing would affect my speaking, but no one ever said that speaking would affect my singing." We worked for several weeks to correct his speaking habits, and then commenced the singing exercises. Your voice can't be free in singing if it isn't free in speaking.

I remember talking with the famous recitalist Roland Hayes many years ago. His speaking voice was so free and resonant that it gave me the feeling that every bone in his body was hollow! The resonance in the recordings of Kirsten Flagstad's speaking voice sounds like a whole orchestra tuning up! Often you hear a person enter a crowded room and greet a friend with such a hearty quality that you say to yourself, "That person must be a singer."

By far, the larger percentage of people I worked with at Barnes Hospital needed help with speaking rather than singing. I had to find a system that could be understood by as large a cross section of patients as possible. The following exercises are very basic, and I found I could adapt them for work with a variety of people. They can be done as a series at one time, or at off moments without special order. The exercises are so simple that their value is often overlooked. Many times, I have had to bring students back to base one after several lessons, because they didn't think they still needed to take time each day with these fundamental exercises.

Exercises for Release

1. Sit in a comfortable, erect position in a straight chair, with your back away from the back of the chair. Let your head fall forward on your chest with its own weight. Then let it swing slowly over as far as your left shoulder, hanging loosely as if falling asleep. Bring your head to an erect position again, then let it fall forward on your chest as before, only this time let it swing slowly to the right shoulder. Bring it to an erect position once more and now let it fall back with your mouth dropping open. With your head hanging back, let it move gently from side to side and then slowly bring it to an erect position once more. Your head should rest as easily on top of your spine as a doll's head balancing on a stick.

(If you have suffered a whiplash, sit in a straight chair placed against a wall, and rest your head against the wall. Keeping contact with the wall, let your head roll to the right with its own weight, then to the left.)

2. Imitate a yawning motion several times. If a real yawn comes, do not stifle it—enjoy it.

3. Check your jaw for looseness. See if you can drop your jaw open and then move it gently up and down and side to side with your hands. If you can't do it immediately, slowly move your jaw up and down and side to side with your jaw muscles, hands following, your thumbs under your chin and fingers above. Then move your hands faster to see if you can catch your jaw muscles off guard. It may take more than one try to do this. A loose jaw helps to induce a loose larynx.

4. Massage the muscles along your jaw in a circular motion with your index fingers under your jaw bone. Include the muscles in the cheeks and extend the motion upward to include the temples and muscles of bite. Massage the muscles under your chin, the hyoglossus and associated muscles. This area should remain soft at all times when singing.

5. Massage the right side of your neck with your left hand against your throat. The thumb will be massaging the left side. Then reverse, with your right hand massaging the left side. Your jaw should hang so loosely that your teeth would click if you flapped your jaw shut in a hurry. When the jaw is relaxed, it drops down and in. Rest your fingers under your chin and jiggle it up and down to help loosen this whole area.

6. Imagine that you are loosely chewing food while speaking. The more sloppy and relaxed, the better. This originates from the Froeschels hypothesis that humans invented language by combining the various sounds they made while eating (Weiss & Beebe, 1951, p. 11). The process of chewing involves a very natural and free motion of the muscles of the jaw, tongue, and pharynx. Avoid clenching your teeth.

7. Take an easy breath and release it like a sigh. Avoid raising your shoulders or chest and maintain your posture as your breath goes out. Repeat until you feel all parts of the body free as you slowly breathe in and let the air out.

8. To release tension in the tongue, let your tongue lie passively in your mouth with the tip resting behind the lower teeth or out over your lower lip. Let your jaw hang open.

9. When practicing sounds later, if the back of your tongue still seems tight, stick it out and hold it with your thumb and fore-finger. A paper towel or handkerchief is necessary so that your tongue will not slip out of your fingers. In this position, starting with an aspirated *h*, lightly sound the *a* as in cat [æ]; the back of your mouth should feel like the beginning of a yawn. Let your voice slide downward with a slightly breathy inflection. If your tongue is pulling back against your fingers, this indicates the area that needs to be released. No matter how high or low you phonate, there should be no pull from the base of your tongue. Use only the vowel [æ] in this exercise. Follow it by humming lightly with your tongue sticking out between your lips.

10. One way to relieve body tension is to stand and stretch, hands over your head, letting your body swing loosely and slowly to the left and right, then back and forward. Let your body bend forward and hang, gently shaking the entire body, neck, shoulders, and arms, Slowly straighten up, erecting your head last.

11. If your whole body feels tense, lie on the floor on your back. Then lazily roll side to side to remind your body of what it could do when you were young.

12. Here's another exercise to induce complete body release. Sit comfortably, with your eyes closed, and, starting from the top of your head, feel that all the muscles of the skull and fore-head are sagging and that all tension is slipping away, being absorbed into the floor (or ground) beneath you—much as moisture condensed on the outside of an iced drink slips down and is absorbed by the napkin beneath. Proceed with the back of your neck, then the temples and sides of the neck, the jaw and cheeks, the shoulders, upper arms, fore-arms, wrists, hands, fingers, then back through the shoulder blades, back, chest, and so on—until you have gone to your toes. It might take five minutes, but it will be one of the most rewarding five minutes you ever spent. Business people sometimes stop, do this for five minutes, and then feel greatly refreshed for continuing their work.

It is important to have your head easily poised with your larynx resting in a relaxed, relatively low position, because the muscles for pitch adjustment work below the Adam's apple. Muscles above are used primarily in chewing and swallowing and should not be active in phonation. Avoid pulling your larynx down.

These exercises should be done at the start of each day before sounds are tried. They can be repeated through the day or they can also be used to unwind after singing. They are essential to creating the conditions under which other muscles can be called into action.

For each action, there is a counterbalancing suppression of action not needed. By thinking, some muscles are activated in preparation for a sound, while others are suppressed. How beautifully nature works for us!

THE MIND–BODY CONNECTION

There is two-way communication between mind and body. If the mind is completely at ease, the message goes to the body that everything is OK, so there is no need for tension. Likewise, if the body is relaxed, a message goes to the mind to stop worrying. Free, easy breathing, as we breathe in sleep, is part of a relaxed body. Breathing easily is the key to bringing about release.

Some interference may require medical diagnosis such as a stiff neck or a malfunctioning disc. Correction could include any of several medical or physical therapy approaches, depending on the finding. Most physicians begin with conservative treatments and find that the desired change can be achieved without invasive measures.

Sometimes you may have difficulty opening and closing your mouth. This may be caused by pressure in the temporal mandibular joint, the point where your jaw is hinged to your skull. A good dentist is usually one of the first to consult if such a problem exists. Great progress is being made in the diagnosis and treatment of this condition.

Many voice students have a tendency to raise one or both shoulders toward the end of a long or intense phrase in singing. By working very hard to control your breathing, as explained in the next chapter, you can usually correct this interfering habit.

A young lady studying with me had just such a habit. On long notes, especially, her right shoulder would rise. One day I tapped her shoulder to remind her of what was happening. To her amazement, when she relaxed her shoulder the note went completely out of tune. By learning to manage her breathing without shoulder interference, she got back on track.

Tuning in to the tensions that interfere with vocal production requires a great deal of concentration. Try to become aware of what has gotten in your way, and practice to bring about release.

Meditation can work wonders as you learn to focus your thinking on particular functions of the body, but it takes time. You must dedicate yourself to whatever routine is necessary to become free both mentally and physically.

The subjects of relaxation, meditation, yoga, and other such techniques have been treated in many books and papers. Both the Alexander (*The Resurrection of the Body*, 1969, NY, NY. University Books.) and Feldenkreis (*Awareness Through Movement*, 1972, NY, NY. Harper & Row.) techniques have great value. Special problems may require exercises and treatments that are beyond the scope of this book. By all means, explore anything that can remove interference.

As you proceed through the next few chapters, you will see how important it is to identify and eliminate points of strain. Chapter XVI, entitled Laryngeal Anatomy and Physiology plus the one on Neurology and the Brain (Chapter XVII) show how other parts of the body influence vocal production. Become aware of tensions in the body that inhibit your freedom of motion and determine how these tensions develop. Often, something as simple as trying too hard can be the difficulty. The harder you try, the less well your voice responds.

Discovering a sense of neutral suspension will better prepare you for the next steps in this book. Use this sense of equilibrium as a reference point. A condition of release serves as the basis for everything that follows.

The better you can *think* at this stage of study, the easier it will be to *let* when the time comes. Since voice responds to the mental concept, you must *think* before you can *let*, and your body must be free to respond.

REFERENCES

Lea & Febiger. (1954). *Gray's anatomy* (26th ed., p. 1087). Philadelphia, Pa: Lea & Febiger.

Weiss, D. A., & Beebe, H. H. (1951). *The chewing approach in speech and voice therapy.* Basel, Switzerland: Karger.

III

■

POSTURE AND BREATHING

The only time I heard Kirsten Flagstad in concert, I was sitting on stage behind her. I couldn't help but notice her breathing. Her back opened and compressed like a huge bellows. After the concert I met a friend who was sitting in row L, center orchestra. "Did you notice her breathing?" she asked, then continued, "I couldn't see a thing move!" I answered, "You should have been where I was. I saw everything!"

Flagstad had learned that the strongest muscle actions we are aware of in singing are those at the sides and back. Ordinarily, the front is where we see the greatest motion because there are no anterior bone structures between the bottom of the ribs and the pelvis. At the sides and back, the distance between the ribs and pelvis is relatively short. During active expiration, the muscles at the sides exert the strongest contractions, blending with those felt at the back; the ones in front take third place. You can check this for yourself by placing your hands at your sides with your fingers back over the area between your pelvis and lower ribs, and then vigorously saying, "Hey!"

Students and teachers of voice have given attention to posture and breathing for thousands of years. One reason is that an efficient and natural supply of air is needed for voice production. Gould (1971) states that voice production can be considered "secondary to the postural mechanism which directly affects respiratory activity." Further, Gould and Okamura (1974) state that "the standard definition of posture is the totality of dynamic inter-relationships between neural, muscular and skeletal elements involved in

17

determining, maintaining and changing not only postural attitudes but also the rate and volume of respiration in regard to the demands of the body's need which includes voice production."

THE DIAPHRAGM AND MUSCLES USED FOR POSTURE

As human beings we must work on good posture because we evolved from a four-legged species. Animals have no problem in keeping their ribs expanded. Babies go through a stage of crawling before they walk. In her book *The Thinking Body*, Mable Todd explains that as an infant develops "active movements and the resultant deeper breathing bring about the coordinated action of the entire spine. This process is greatly aided by spells of crying and screaming, since the diaphragm and the lower lumbar and pelvic muscles are so closely associated" (1937, pp. 94, 251). You can see, then, how nature integrates the body as we are growing and prepares us for the connection of posture and breathing for voice use.

Much emphasis has been placed on the action of the diaphragm in breathing. To gain a proper understanding of how the diaphragm functions, it is important to know that its motion is influenced by posture. *Gray's Anatomy* tells us that our diaphragm "stands highest when the body is horizontal and the patient on his back, and in this position it performs the largest respiratory excursions with normal breathing" (Lea & Febiger, 1954, p. 456)

The part of the spine that is most flexible is the lumbar region —that section between the ribs and the pelvis (Figure III–1). Watch a good belly dancer and you'll see just how flexible it is! The strongest muscles for breathing are attached to the inner surfaces of that lumbar spine.

To breathe freely, the body needs good alignment. Notice in Figure III–1 how near the anterior portion of the lumbar vertebrae come to the middle of your body. The crura, the longest fibers of the diaphragm, are attached to the innermost portion of the first three lumbar vertebrae. If the curvature of the spine is too great, the crura would be elongated and not able to exert their optimal contraction. In the same area, the psoas major and psoas minor attach to the sides of all the lumbar vertebrae and extend to the pelvis and thigh (Figure III–2). They are strong postural muscles and assist in counteracting any excess curvature of the spine. Because of the location of these muscles, it has not been possible to measure the exact extent of their activity.

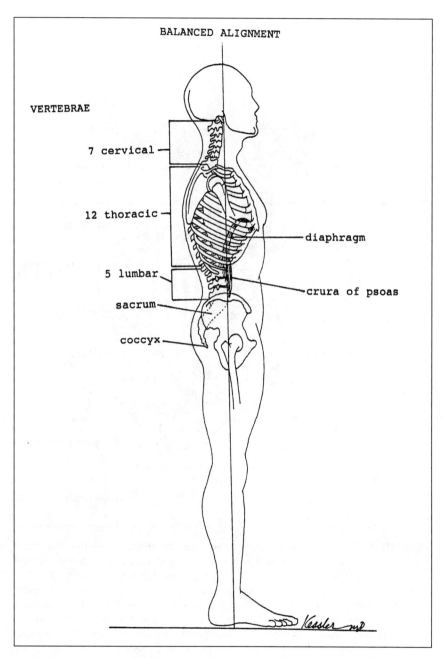

Figure III–1. Balanced alignment. Note how the vertebrae are related to the midline. The arch of the diaphragm from inside the sternum to the anterior of the lumbar vertebrae is also shown. Also note the crura.

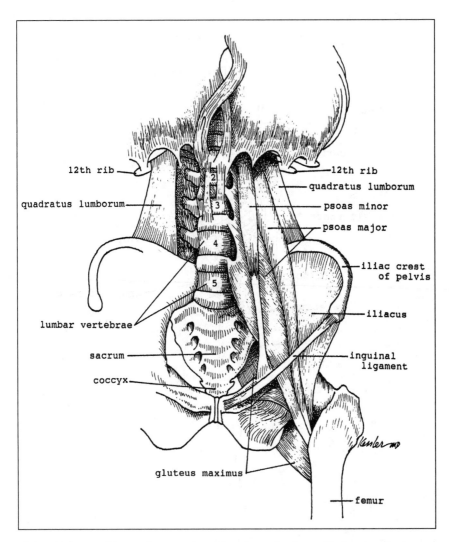

Figure III–2. Tucking-under muscles. View from the front. Under the diaphragm above, the psoas minor and psoas major extend downward from their lateral attachments to the 12th thoracic and all of the lumbar vertebrae over the iliac crest, the psoas major going all the way to the femur. The gluteus maximum extends posteriorly from the pelvis down to the inferior sides of the sacrum, coccyx, and the femur. All relate to the power humans have of maintaining the trunk in an erect posture. By their downward pull, they counterbalance the upward pull of the muscles in Figure III–3a. The quadratus lumborum contributes to the firmness felt in the small of the back.

One way to become aware of body alignment is to develop your sixth sense. For a long time I didn't know there was such a thing, but it has a name: *proprioception*. A proprioceptor is a sensory receptor (nerve ending) that responds to stimuli from muscles, tendons, ligaments, and joints. This can give a "perceiving of self." It tells of movement in all skeletal and muscular structures. Scientists call it *kinesthesia*. In addition to developing your kinesthetic sensibilities, you can study the alignment of your body in a mirror. A three-way mirror such as you find in a clothing store is, of course, the best for this. Another way is to use a hand mirror together with a full-length mirror to see whether your posture needs special attention. A video camera will catch both posture and sound.

EXERCISES FOR GOOD POSTURE

Here are some exercises to help you develop good posture:

1. Lie on your back on the floor. At the outset, you will notice a space between the small of your back and the floor, but eventually your spine will relax enough to almost touch the floor at all points. A small space is normal. Is there extra space? If so, raise your knees so that your feet are flat on the floor. Rotate your pelvis as if lengthening it away from your head. At the same time, let the back of your neck elongate away from the torso, chin "in" without forcing, as if you are trying to see your toes. Raise your arms over your head, and rest them on the floor. These actions tend to elongate the spine. Rest in this position for a short time, letting gravity help to settle your limbs and torso into a relaxed condition. After at least five minutes, notice how your breathing behaves. There should be an easy ebb and flow just below the ribs.

2. When your body has accustomed itself to this position, gradually slide your feet forward one leg at a time until your legs are straight. Maintain the elongated position of the spine. Slowly bring your arms to your sides again, one at a time. Try to keep the space small between your spine and the floor. When your legs are fully extended, again let your body get accustomed to the position for several minutes. Breathe easily. In this position, notice that your rib cage is considerably expanded.

3. As you gain a sense of what the alignment of your body feels like from head to toe, then stand by rolling to one side, bring up your knees, and thus bring your body weight over your legs. Feel you are standing tall with the floor still behind you. Standing tall helps to elevate your rib cage and corresponds to the position your ribs were in when you were lying on the floor.

4. In a standing position, place your hands at your sides, thumbs forward with fingers extending back between the bottom of your ribs and top of your pelvis. Let your head hang loosely forward. Bend your knees without lifting your heels off the floor. You should feel an expansion in your back under your fingers. Now slowly straighten your legs, keeping the back expanded. You will notice that your lower abdominal wall draws in. Slowly bring your head to an erect position. You now find that your chest is expanded. If you have not tried to control your breathing, you will discover that the upper abdominal area between your "belt line" and bottom ribs moves freely in and out with each breath. Try to avoid any tension at the front of your neck.

5. Continue standing tall as if you were trying to touch something above with the top of your head. Another thought is to pretend you are being suspended from above like a puppet dangling on a string. If you can maintain a mental image of being tall but loose, you will gradually develop awareness of how your head rests on top of the spine, the neck rests between the shoulders, the ribs float out from the upper part of the back, the torso sits into the pelvis, the pelvis rests on the legs, and the feet and toes feel rooted to the floor.

6. Perhaps you have heard the expression "pinching a penny between the buttocks." It is a useful image. With this alignment in place, see if your breath is still taking care of itself in an easy ebb and flow between your ribs and the lower abdominal area. These lower abdominal muscles should be firm, which is brought about in part by activating the transversalis muscle (Figure III–3a, b, c). This firmness aids in supporting the visceral organs. It functions to create a firm foundation for the breathing action which takes place above it. This aspect of posture is readily observable in ballet dancers, who keep the lower abdominal area firm, but allow the upper part to be free for breathing and movement. The buttocks should be tucked under (Figure III–2)

7. To help firm the lower abdominal muscles, either lie on your back on the floor or sit forward on the edge of a chair. With your legs straight, raise your feet a few inches. While holding

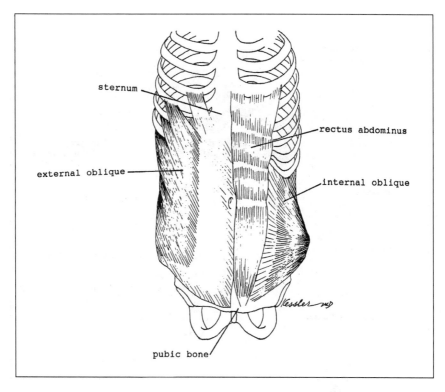

Figure III–3a. Abdominal muscles—front view. The external oblique, internal oblique, and the rectus abdominus tend to draw the pubic bone toward the sternum and thus to elongate the spine while holding the viscera firm.

your feet up, spread them apart,then bring them together again and slowly let them return to the floor. Keep your throat open and breathe easily during the exercise. Repeat several times.

8. While standing, let your body weight be slightly forward on the balls of your feet. A certain freedom is gained in having the weight forward rather than on your heels. To test this, concentrate on how the muscles in your torso and neck feel as you first let the weight of your body rest back on your heels and then let your body move slightly forward over the balls of your feet. You will notice that the muscles at the front of your body stiffen slightly when your weight is over your heels. By comparison, they are more relaxed when

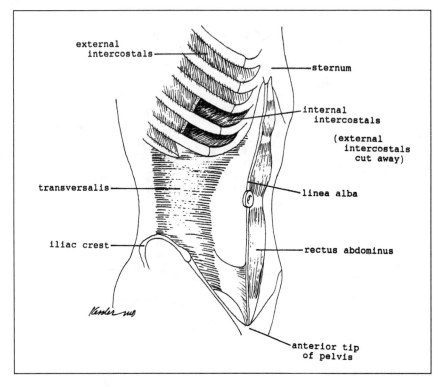

Figure III–3b. Right side. The transversalis muscles act with the above to oppose the lowering of the diaphragm and to compress the viscera. This creates a maximum of compression for control of the expiration of air. The external and internal intercostal muscles are shown above.

your weight is forward. This is particularly important as it applies to the front of your neck and throat.

9. Now see if you can walk with this very tall bearing. Feel free movement at the knee joint. As an experiment, take ten steps, paying attention to how your whole body feels. Then let your body go back to your accustomed way of standing and repeat those ten steps. Did you feel heavier than when you were keeping yourself tall? Look at yourself in a mirror and be honest: Isn't the tall posture pretty good to look at? Doesn't it give you a sense of well-being?

A tall young man just out of high school came to me for study. He was a good example of the lanky boy who grew much

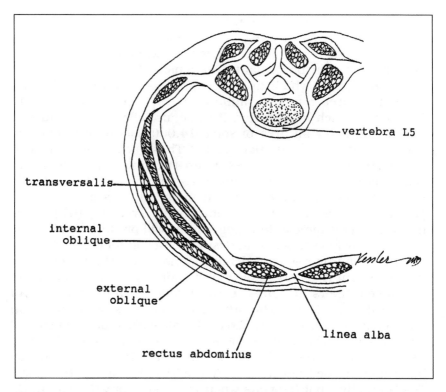

Figure III–3c. From above—right side. A cross section of the body at the level of the 5th lumbar vertebrae.

faster than his classmates and stooped to conceal his height. We worked on his stooping posture through the year, with no apparent result—at least, I had to constantly remind him. The next year when he returned to school I exclaimed, "You've grown taller through the summer." He answered, "No. I just stretched out what I had!" The new bearing was finally there to stay and it was great. I say, if you're tall, be gloriously tall, but don't try to be taller than you are.

THE DIAPHRAGM AND MUSCLES USED FOR BREATHING

Now let's take a look at breathing. Richard Cone (1908) states that the practice which must precede all others is the method of taking a breath.

A few facts about the lungs will help you realize how much they can do for you. To give yourself an image, compare the lungs to a tree upside down. The trunk is your windpipe, and the large branches are your bronchial tubes. Smaller branches lead to the twigs and leaves which are your air cells. Each of us has an estimated three hundred million air cells measuring 1/70 to 1/200 of an inch in diameter. If these air cells were spread out, they would cover an area of some 14,000 square feet—close to one-third of an acre (Kofler, 1887)! These cells are lined with elastic tissue that stretches when the lungs are filled and contracts when you stop inhaling. A supply of air is needed to produce tone. You take a breath in but it goes out by itself, passively, doing the work for you. Donald Proctor (1979) states that this elastic force at full lung volume will produce a subglottic pressure "far in excess of that desired for a soft tone" (p. 31).

The diaphragm is considered the most important muscle for breathing, but it is impossible to put your finger on it. One end of its muscle fibers attaches to the inside of the lower ribs all around (Figure III–4a). The other end converges on a tendon in the middle of your body. Relaxed, the muscles appear something like an inverted bowl. When activated, the muscles shorten and the center is lowered (Figure III–4b). If I held a balloon in my hand and pressed down on it, it would bulge out at the sides. That's exactly what happens when you take a breath—you bulge out at the sides.

In filling the lungs some of the body's weight has been lifted against gravity. When the inspiratory muscles are relaxed, gravity tends to bring the weight down again. Also, ligamentous attachments have been stretched and their recoil assists in bringing the chest back to a position of rest. The abdominal muscles, which also have been stretched, have an elastic property which helps return them to their original position.

Several other actions occur when the diaphragm moves downward. If your lower abdomen is firm, the diaphragm tends to exert a lateral pressure which assists in expanding the lower ribs (Watson & Hixon, 1985). More important, it helps to lower and widen the glottal opening in your throat. There is an explanation for this, described by Zemlin (1984) in an article in the *National Association of Teachers of Singing Bulletin*:

> The pericardium is a fibro-serous sack in which the heart and the roots of the great vessels are contained. At the very top are fibers which have an attachment to the larynx. Below,

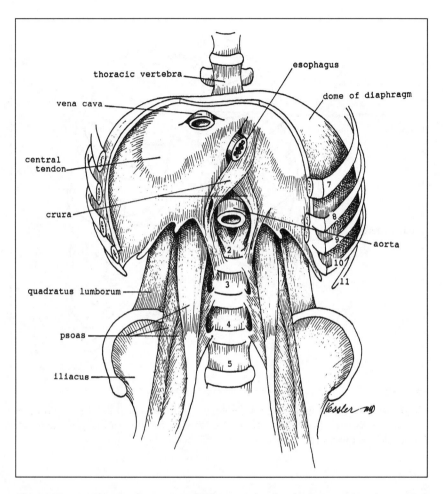

Figure III–4a. The diaphragm. Looking up under the front, exposing the central tendon. The crura and psoas both have attachments to the interior portion of the lumbar vertebrae.

the pericardium blends into and contributes to the central portion of the diaphragm. It is therefore reasonable to expect abrupt and strong contractions of the diaphragm musculature to influence the position of the larynx. There will be a descent of the larynx with a quick deep breath. (p. 4)

Your rib cage is expanded by the *external intercostal* muscles and contracted by the internal intercostals (see Figure III–3b).

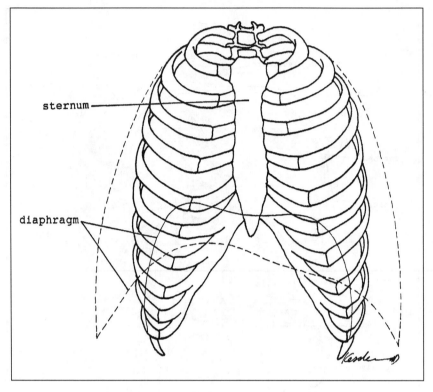

Figure III–4b. Outline of ribs and diaphragm from the front. Solid line shows the diaphragm at rest. Broken line shows the lowered position of the diaphragm and expansion of the rib cage on inspiration.

When your ribs expand, you have the greatest mechanical advantages to support phonation (Baker, 1979). This is important. Have you ever seen an opera singer with a collapsed chest?

NATURAL BREATHING

The following are some experiments to illustrate how nature fills your lungs. Keep a good posture while trying them. First, place one hand on your chest and the other under your ribs. This will help make you aware of what is happening. While standing tall, keep your rib cage expanded but not pulled up.

1. a. Empty your lungs completely while maintaining your posture.
   b. Don't let any air into your lungs until your system needs oxygen.
   c. When you need air, let it go where it wants to. Where did you feel the motion—under your upper or lower hand? Most people say the lower.

2. Stand with your hands positioned as before. Empty your lungs completely, but this time suddenly open your mouth and let the air go where it wants. Again, expansion is felt primarily under the lower hand.

3. With hands and stance as before, sniff as if you smelled something burning. You should feel quick motions in the abdominal area below your ribs.

The diaphragm acts on the lungs much as the piston in a gas engine draws gas into the cylinder. The contraction of the diaphragm creates a negative pressure in the lungs above. As air comes in, it fills the tiny air sacs with oxygen in exchange for carbon dioxide, which is expelled on expiration. Expanding your rib cage tends to pull the attached fibers of the diaphragm outward, and thus also assists in lowering the diaphragm when you fill your lungs.

Some people have difficulty feeling the slightly outward movement in their backs induced by taking a breath (see Figure III–2). One way to increase awareness is to bend forward while sitting in a straight chair. With your fingers extended over the small of your back, take a full breath. After observing the expansion several times, raise your body a little and repeat. In stages, come to a straight sitting position. You should still be aware of the outward motion in your back when taking a breath. Finally, try to feel this same motion when standing.

An oversimplification of the flow of air in and out of the lungs would be to compare it to the swing of a pendulum. Starting with the pendulum at the point of full swing, let this represent the full expansion of your lungs. If you do not hold the "inspiratory muscles," the air goes out—just as the pendulum will drop and swing to the opposite side if you let go of it. This now represents the lungs when empty. If you relax all expiratory forces, the air will again rush in to fill the vacuum, just as the pendulum will swing back to its original full swing position. The idea is to relax the inspiratory muscles for expiration and relax the expiratory muscles for inspiration, all within the framework of good posture. Despite the oversimplification, the imagery has the virtue of removing unnecessary effort in terms of how one should breathe.

Some time ago, in checking the breathing of a new student, I asked him to take a comfortably full breath. In doing so he distended his lower abdomen so much that he looked pregnant. I asked him why he did this and he replied that his teacher had told him that this was the way to get a "low" breath. I explained that "low" means not to heave with his shoulders and chest. To allow your lower abdomen to protrude as he did is to completely lose all possibility of securing a firm foundation for the action of the muscles above. Being soft, the viscera need to be contained by the abdominal muscles to provide a solid base against which the diaphragm can create a full compression.

RELATIONSHIP BETWEEN BREATHING AND SINGING

To help understand the capacity of the lungs in breathing, I include an illustration of the various volume levels (Figure III–5). In singing, the vital capacity should be used. This means taking a comfortably full breath, not a strained expansion. The breathing potential is divided into several levels. The *tidal volume* is what is used in normal, easy breathing. If you take as full a breath as possible, you have filled the area called *complemental volume*. If you expel as much air as possible, you have reached into the *supplemental volume*. *Residual volume* is what is left in your lungs when you have expelled as much air as possible. *Vital capacity* uses the full range of volume above residual volume. Having sufficient breath for singing is not related to lung capacity. Singers do not necessarily have greater lung capacity, but they are much more efficient at utilizing the air stored in their lungs.

In moments of compressed expiration, the muscles that attach to the lower part of the pelvis (tucking under) are the true foundation (see Figure III–2). Without this fixative action, those abdominal muscles which extend from the upper posterior surface of the pelvis to the lower ribs would not have a firm base to provide the energy needed for long phrases or dramatic singing. Flagstad is reported to have said that her legs got tired after long periods of singing, but not her throat. This experience in deep connection to breathing usually comes only when voices are fully matured. Practicing the exercises for posture and breathing prepares the way.

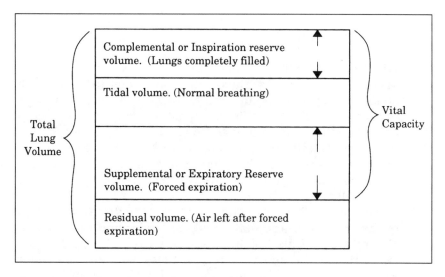

Figure III–5. Volume levels in lungs during breathing.

BREATHING EXERCISES

The exercises that were given for posture at the beginning of this chapter should have established a relatively expanded chest for breathing. Let your shoulders remain calm and relaxed. When short of breath after running, your shoulders provide an assisting action. For singing, you definitely don't want to give the impression of being in a state of "emergency."

Breathing exercises are designed to bring reflexive action under cortical control so that it will be ready and responsive to the demands of singing. As you do the exercises, breathe in through your nose. It is nature's own filtering, heating, and humidifying system. "Catch breaths" are taken through your mouth, of course. These belong where there are only short rests or no rests at all. They tend to dry your mouth and throat, however. Proper lubrication of your vocal folds is very important. Breathing through your nose whenever you have time provides essential moisture.

1. Slowly fill your lungs over a 10-second span, reaching full capacity at 10. Exhale through pursed lips; lungs empty at

10. Gradually increase to 11 seconds, then 12, and so on. If you get to 20, that's probably far enough. Go only as far as you can go comfortably.

2. With separate sniffs at each step, either while out walking briskly or walking in place, fill your lungs in four quick sniffs—one each step—and empty them in the next four steps in separate puffs. Maintain your posture. Vary the number of impulse patterns from time to time, such as: in 6, out 6; in 8, out 8; in 20, out 20; in 2, out 10; in 1, out 10; in 3, out 2, and so on. Keep your shoulders relaxed and your chest relatively calm. As a student, I used to constantly practice this while walking.

3. Elevate your rib cage *without taking a breath* by the action of the external intercostals. Keep shoulder and throat muscles relaxed. While holding your ribs expanded and throat open, repeat the above exercises. Relax your rib cage after each exercise; then, elevate again and try a different one.

4. Here are a series of exercises to strengthen and develop awareness of your intercostals and your diaphragm. All should be undertaken in the healthy posture described earlier in this chapter.

A. 1. Raise your chest without taking a breath.
   2. Take a deep breath and hold it with diaphragm.
   3. Keep your throat open and relaxed, extend your arms to sides with your palms forward.
   4. With your arm muscles tense, slowly flex your arms at the elbow until your fingers touch your chest.
   5. Straighten your arms, then drop them to your sides.
   6. Expel air, keeping your chest expanded.
   7. Relax your chest and rest a bit.

B. 1. Repeat steps A.1 through A.3, but with your palms up.
   4. With your arm muscles tense, slowly flex your elbows, bringing your fingers to your shoulders.
   5. Straighten your arms and drop them to your sides.
   6. Expel air, keeping your chest expanded.
   7. Relax your chest.

C. 1. Repeat A.1 and A.2.
   3. Leaving your arms at your sides, point your palms forward.
   4. Flexing at the elbows, slowly bring your fingers to your shoulders as though you were lifting a heavy weight.
   5. Drop arms to your sides again.

6. Expel air, keeping your chest expanded.
7. Relax your chest.

D. 1. Repeat steps A.1 and A.2
   3. Place the palms of your hands together as if in prayer.
   4. Shoot arms upward and then swing them down sideways with a slight backwards movement in an arc.
   5. Reverse this gesture, returning your hands to the prayer pose.
   6. Expel air, keeping your chest expanded.
   7. Relax your chest.

This series of exercises (A–D) is from the book *Voice Building and Tone Placement*, by H. Holbrook Curtis, first published in 1896 (p. 213). The exercises are vigorous, so you should limit yourself to A and B for a few days. Gradually, C and D can be added. Do them only once at each practice session.

5. This exercise will help bring your breathing under cortical control. Lie on the floor in the position established for good posture. Notice how your breath flows in and out in an easy, relaxed manner. To be conscious of this, place one hand on your chest and the other just below your ribs. Now imagine the music is in 4/4 time and that you need to start singing on "1" of the second measure. Count the beats in seconds. Time your inspiration to be ready to phonate on "1" of the second measure. Your breath should be taken with the same natural motion of expansion in the abdominal area as has been observed in the quiet breathing above. The purpose of practicing this kind of exercise is to establish a means of inhaling with the least effort at a particular point in time. Pace this so that you release air on "1" without holding at "4."

6. To illustrate how an expiratory flow of air will automatically produce a sound:
  a. Form your teeth and lips for a hissing sound (Hssss).
  b. Take a breath and release the air through this resistance on count "1." Try to feel what is happening inside your body during this expiration. At first, you might think you are pushing air out. On further investigation, however, you will become aware of a pressure or compression taking place inside the thoracic cage. It is this pressure that many people refer to as "breath support." Learn to think in terms of breath pressure or compression rather than "support."

Obviously, the muscles referred to in the text and illustrations are only a few of the more important ones involved in posture and breathing. For greater detail, it would be necessary to examine such books as *Gray's Anatomy* (1954); Zemlin's *Speech and Hearing Science* (1968); Bunch's *Dynamics of the Singing Voice* (1982); and others.

MAINTAINING AIR PRESSURE AND BREATH CONTROL

There is a law in physics known as the *Venturi effect* (see Chapter XV). Think of what happens to a garden hose when you narrow the nozzle so that water will reach a distant point. The pressure from the source of water—a lake or water tower—is now pushing against the circumference of the hose because of a back pressure created by the narrowing of the nozzle. When the nozzle is opened, the pressure along the body of the hose is relieved and water runs freely from the nozzle. All this time, however, the water pressure at the source has been constant.

In the same way, the varied conditions at the glottis can affect the amount of compression within the lungs. Our lungs are like the lake or water tower and have a full supply of energy available as soon as we take a breath. In phonation, the glottis acts as the point of resistance like the nozzle on the hose.

To quote Lilli Lehman (1909): "We first become conscious of the vocal cords through the controlling apparatus of the breath, which teaches us to spare them, by emitting breath through them in the least possible quantity and of even pressure, whereby a steady tone can be produced. I even maintain that all is won, when—as Victor Maurel says—we regard them directly as the breath regulators and relieve them of all overwork through the controlling apparatus of the chest-muscle tension" (p. 25).

During phonation, a considerable degree of activity takes place in the diaphragm in opposition to the forces working to expel air when a sound is initiated. This acts as a control in establishing the desired compression for the tone. Leanderson and Sundberg explain this in great detail in their article "Breathing for Singing." Incidentally, it interested me to learn that a race car driver keeps one foot ready on the brake while the other is on the throttle. It is this attention to opposing forces that gives control.

When the great tenor Beniamino Gigli was asked what he did for breath support, he answered, "I take a breath." Trust that the energy will be there when you need it and you will never have to worry about the mystery of supporting a tone. Breath will connect with the tone and the release of air will do the work. Eventually, you will feel "compression" or firmness in the abdominal area, with an especially taut feeling in the lower half of the abdomen. In time, this spreads very strongly into the lower back and even into the buttocks and thighs. Don't try for it. You will find it happening when the right time comes.

Luciano Pavarotti once confided to me, "Meester Brown, eet's like-a you go to the bathroom!" After testing his words of wisdom in the lavatory, I discovered that what he must have meant was that it is like you need to go to the bathroom—only you find that someone else is already there, so you must wait—!?*! When this happens, a low compression is created. There is no need for tension in the laryngeal area, however.

William Vennard (1967) has stated that breath control should not be taught until a free flowing tone is mastered. It is a matter of *breath management,* not *breath control* (p. 34). I concur with this and teach breathing exercises to be practiced independently from tone production! This develops an awareness of what the breath can do so that it will be ready to connect to tone when the time comes.

I have heard Friedrich Brodnitz say, "The goal of good singing can best be reached with the greatest economy of air." The trained, reflexive action will do the work. When the laryngeal muscles have become sufficiently conditioned, it is as if the larynx were reaching down for, or drawing on, the energy that is there by nature through proper inspiration, but this can only take place through development over a period of time. It is then that you begin to understand what Proctor (1979) meant when he stated that "the beautiful voice is the result not of exertion of great power but rather of delicate control" (p. 14).

IMPROVING POSTURE AND BREATHING

There are many schools of thought for improving posture and breathing. One of the oldest is the practice of yoga. There are those who find great benefit from the Alexander Technique, as well as from Feldenkreis, who studied with F. M. Alexander at one time. Another valuable source is *Breathing, the ABC's* by Carola H. Speads (1978). The exercises suggested in this chapter are by no means all there is to know on the subject.

It takes great dedication over a long period of time to practice breathing separately from singing and then gradually discover how it is coordinated with tone production. The rewards are great, however. If proper coordination is not achieved, you have to keep going back in your training to establish these fundamentals for efficient singing.

Thinking is necessary to create the proper conditions. If you have trained your *thinking* and done your practice, you can *trust* the result if you will just *let* it happen.

REFERENCES

Baken, R.J., & Cavallo, M.S. (1979). Chest wall preparation, in *Transcripts of the 8th Symposium*, Care of the professional voice, Part II (pp.19–24). New York: The Voice Foundation.

Cone, R.W. (1908). *The speaking voice* (p. 29). Boston: Evans Music Co.

Curtis, H.H. (1973). *Voice building and tone placement*, Minneapolis, MN: Pro Musical Press. (Reprinted 1909, New York: D. Appleton, 3rd ed.) (Originally published 1896.)

Gould, W.J. (1971). *Effect of respiratory and postural mechanisms upon action of the vocal folds*, Folia Phoniatrica, 23, pp. 211–224.

Gould, W.J. & Okamura, H. (1974). *Respiratory training of the singer*, Folia Phoniatrica, 26, pp. 275–286.

Gray, H. (1954). *Anatomy of the human body*, Philadelphia: Lea & Febiger, p. 456.

Kofler, L. (1887). *The art of breathing*, New York: Edgar S. Werner, p. 31.

Leanderson, R. & Sundberg, J. (1988). *Breathing for singing*, in Journal of Voice, 2 (1), New York: Raven Press, p. 2.

Lehman, L. (1909). *How to sing* (Richard Aldrich, trans.) New York, Macmillan, p. 25.

Proctor, D.F. (1979). *Breath, the power source of the voice*, in Transcripts of the 8th Symposium, Care of the professional voice, Part II, New York: The Voice Foundation, p. 14.

Speads, C. (1978). *Breathing, the ABC's*, New York: Harper & Row.

Todd, M. (1937). *The thinking body*, New York: Dance Horizons, pp. 94, 251.

Vennard, W. (1967). *Singing, the mechanism and the technic*, New York: Carl Fischer, p. 34.

Watson, P.J. & Hixon, T. (1985). *Respiratory kinematics in classical (Opera) singers*, in Journal of Speech and Hearing Research, 28, pp. 104–122.

Zemlin, W.R. (1984). *Notes on the morphology of the human larynx*, in National Association of Teachers of Singing Bulletin, vol. 41, (1), p. 4.

IV

■

ELICITING PITCHES: BEGINNING EXERCISES

In Chapter I, you met Celia, who added, after her glorious burst of primal sound, "But I can't just let my voice go off like that, not knowing what's going to happen, not controlling it!"

"That's *exactly* what I do want you to do!" I said. Subsequently, I told her this story: I had a dream that I was floating through space. I had no fear. Indeed, it was a delicious experience, floating without effort, completely detached. Eventually—alas!—I woke up and found myself on the floor. I'd been gradually slipping off the edge of my bed.

This is the fate Celia feared for her voice. So I told her about Skip, my son-in-law, who recently completed his 1,000th parachute jump. When I first expressed anxiety about his safety, he laughed:

"There's nothing to it! You just float out there in the sky, turn left or right, go with or into the wind."

"And how do you do that?" I asked.

"Oh, we have been trained and conditioned in what to expect."

That's the big difference between my dream and Skip's parachuting experience; Skip had been trained.

Let's use these two experiences as metaphors for the two functions of the larynx for making sound. My dream might be compared to phonation that is involuntary and Skip's parachute jumping to phonation that is voluntary.

Skip told me that sky divers receive a minimum of eight hours of instruction and then must pass a written test before they are allowed to jump. Each jumper has a reserve canopy, or "chute." The reserve chute opens automatically if the jumper is descending at a certain rate at 1,000 feet above ground level. Before each jump, a sky diver adjusts his altimeter to the barometric ground level pressure where he plans to jump.

That's the big difference between the floating of a parachute and the floating of a singing tone. The singer has no "reserve canopy." The singer's only protection against failure is thorough preparation. This means learning how and what to think. A free release of tone in singing gives the sensation that the tone is floating, yet it will respond to thought. Many students have said that they felt they had no control over the sound when it was properly produced. Our considerations of primal sound, release, posture, and breathing have prepared us for this new experience of letting the voice respond to a thought and a flow of air. Our voice will show us what it can do for us, rather than our pushing to make it do anything. The key words here are *think, let,* and *trust.*

Here's an interesting remark from a sky diver: "Unlike those sports where you have to grit your teeth and go for it, skydiving is just the opposite. In order to excel you have to concentrate on relaxing, being calm and smooth. It's so hard not to try. But once you get your wings (learn to fly without thinking—just like walking) it's the greatest feeling in the world, a sense of real accomplishment."

RELAXING MUSCLES AND ELICITING PITCH

A scientist thinks in terms of *frequency,* which is heard as pitch. To a singer, pitch and frequency are synonymous. *Elicit,* "to draw forth or bring out (something latent or potential)" (Merriam-Webster, 1981) exactly fits the process by which a sound begins. Because you condition the primal sound to respond to a mental concept, a proper concept is crucial. Trust that your vocal folds will adjust automatically. Remember the experience of the student with the flexible fiberscope (Chapter I).

There are two opposing energies in producing sound—the activator and the vibrator. They must act in coordination, so that neither one puts undue stress on the other. In vocal production, *less* is *more.* We seek an approach that allows all functions to be carried out with the least amount of effort for the desired result. This by no means implies that singing does not require energy. Vitality of tone, "concentration," or "focus" are the desired results. Research has demonstrated, however, that there is fuller resonance and stronger tone, when muscles are relaxed (Sundberg, 1974).

If you feel that your larynx is in a low, relaxed position just before you finish taking a breath, then it is ready to initiate the tone. If you wait until you have finished taking a breath, hold it, and then start the tone, you will lose the feeling of keeping the ribs expanded with a low, open larynx, which is important for the correct balance of glottal resistance to air flow. The sensation should be that you almost start to sing before you finish taking a breath.

Start a gentle expiration of air as in a silent *h*. Then let a sound come in. This will produce the primal sound *huh*. If you think a definite pitch at the same time, that pitch will be produced. It's that easy. As you listen to a pitch, the vocal folds automatically adjust to that pitch (Wyke, 1979).

THE EFFORTLESS RELEASE OF SOUND

It will help to review the experiment of taking a breath and releasing a hissing sound (Chapter III, Breathing Exercise No. 6). Next, repeat the primal sounds laid out in the first chapter: *uh huh*, as in yes; *huh*, as in a question; and *huh huh*, as in an easy laugh. These sounds should be neither soft nor loud. Try them over a variety of highs and lows but with no definite pitches. Allow your tongue and jaw to remain passive, your neck and shoulders relaxed. If a free sound is produced, you are on your way.

This is not the full-blown, cultivated voice that comes with practice, but the normal, spontaneous, human sound, free of all effort to "do" anything. Your primal sound is taken in the direction of singing (beyond speech) by the prolongation of a single sound. Thus, you are carrying an involuntary response over into a voluntary action.

SLIDING YOUR VOICE DOWN THE SCALE

Release a sighing sound from high to low several times. Then sound a note in an easy middle range such as A or A-flat plus a note 5 diatonic tones lower as a target. This is a major fifth from 5 to 1. (Exercise I; from here on, the exercises referred to are contained in the appendix for singing exercises. They are also illustrated on the CD and are numbered correspondingly.) Let your voice slide from high to low in the same manner you have just been doing without pitches. The way the voice responds should be exactly the same with or without definite pitch.

At this point, many students tend to set their throat muscles as if the act of singing were different from sighing. I often ask them to stop singing and just release the sound as they did when no pitches were introduced. This is very important. The only difference is adding thought of pitch, and we now know that a thought will bring about an automatic adjustment of the vocal folds.

When you have found you can do this, try sliding your voice an octave from high to low (8 to 1). Perhaps starting from C, the next beginning note would be B, then B-flat, in a descending sequence of half steps (Exercise II). There should be no effort to "make" the lower tone. If it doesn't come easily, don't push. When you have reached a low note comfortably, start the sequence again from a bit higher pitch, perhaps D, then D-flat, and so on. These sounds should always be made easily without thoughts of soft or loud. Just let them happen.

A valuable exercise to ensure a free glottal action is to use the vibrated lips (the "lip trill," as it is called by some) or the Italian rolled r [r]. Start without sound, and then add sound while the lips or tongue continue to vibrate. The focal point of breath pressure should stay at the lips or tongue. Start with the unvoiced [p] for the lips or [t] for the tongue ("ppppp" or "trrrrr"). Your throat muscles should be loose enough to allow a flow of air to keep the tip of the tongue or the lips vibrating. If your throat tightens, the vibration at the lips or tongue will stop. This exercise should be done as gently as possible, lips or tongue loose, with no forced air.

I learned this exercise many years ago from a patient whose throat was so tight that no tone would come out without force. In desperation one day he said, "pppp!"—out flowed a sound. I have found since that similar exercises have been used elsewhere, but I have no idea where they started as an exercise for relaxing the glottal closure.

Another exercise is to blow gently on the edge of a piece of paper held vertically against the lips, while sounding an "oo" vowel [u]. The paper should make a buzzing sound. If the paper stops buzzing, it is because the larynx is too tight to let an easy flow of air through. This exercise was shown to me by Bruce Foote, who headed the Voice Department at the University of Illinois for many years.

If none of these exercises seem to work, try releasing a hissing sound and lightly changing it to z, "sssssssszzzzz." Done at first in descending, sighing inflections, these devices can later be used on scales to ensure a feeling of freedom at the glottis. The term *glottis* refers to the vocal folds and the space between them.

Letting tones slide from top to bottom seems too easy to be called singing, but it is at the very roots of all the training that follows. You are conditioning responses. You are developing a kinesthetic chain of action, which will give you the freedom to focus on the meaning of text and musical values later on.

Next, think of the notes that move 5-4-3-2-1 and let your voice almost slide through each step without special emphasis on each note. Repeat in downward sequences within a comfortable range. Then start at a higher pitch and again progress downward. (Exercise III). Allow the first sound to start lightly each time and relax into a bit fuller tone at the bottom, like a sigh.

Now let the notes of a diatonic major scale come in as you descend just by lazily thinking them: 8-7-6-5-4-3-2-1. Try to avoid accenting each pitch. Remember to go only as low as your voice will produce the notes easily (Exercise IV).

The schwa sound *uh* [ə] is used in these exercises because we probably use fewer muscular adjustments in its formation than with any other vowel sound in any language. If the lips are closed, the humming sound produced will be the *m* [m] hum. Some people move their tongue when they close their mouth producing *ng* [ŋ] or an *n* [n] hum. In *ng*, the back of the tongue rises against the soft palate and prevents the tone from entering the mouth. The *n* hum is produced by raising the front of the tongue against the alveolar ridge, which prevents the tone from reaching the lips. To test for a pure *m* hum, pluck your lower lip with your finger while humming. The sound *uh* [ə] should come out. This shows that the blade of the tongue is resting passively in the mouth with the tip behind the lower teeth.

Return to the experiments in releasing a free tone. After you have established the feeling of connecting an airflow to the production of sound, [ssss], substitute an *m* [m] or the *huh* [hu] for the hissing. Follow the same pattern of a falling inflection. In the *m* hum, the air will start flowing gently through your nose first.

A childlike concept of sound should be used. As you try these exercises, it is important that you feel you are the most agreeable person ever born. Ideally, there should be a feeling of complete release.

SLIDING YOUR VOICE UP THE SCALE

Eventually you must learn how to let notes flow in an upward progression as well. As a starter, try the following (Exercise V). As your voice goes down the scale and up again, feel that the tone bounces on the lower note and then floats lightly back through the tone it started on. It's much like a roller coaster which starts from the highest point and then is carried over the next high peak by momentum. Playing with a yo-yo is another illustration. Once the first note has been properly elicited, a sense of what that frequency feels like is being conditioned. The return to it is a reversal of the first downward motion. Here, we are establishing kinesthetic actions to bring about automatic responses.

ALTERING THE SHAPE OF YOUR SOUND

Explore the use of other vowel sounds. Language is shape. The part of language used for vocalizing is the vowel. Vowels should be formed as easily as possible to ensure free phonation. This subject is taken up in detail in Chapter X on Articulation. For now, if you think of forming the vowels in as simple and childlike a manner as possible, you will probably find a useful shape. Looseness and freedom are more important than a definitive vowel color.

By maintaining the free, open sense of the primal sound *uh* [ə] as the basis for phonation, you should be able to form such vowels as *oo* [u], *o* [o], *ah* [ɑ], *a* [e] and *e* [i]. These are the primary "Italian" vowels. The [u] and [o] are lip vowels and the [e] and [i] are tongue vowels. A metaphor that I have found helpful is to imagine that the schwa *uh* [ə] is like a spotlight at the back of the throat, there as part of every vowel. The shapes needed for other vowels might then be compared to colored gelatins in front of the spotlight altering the value of the sound that reaches our ears. Thinking about it this way helps to keep a free, open feeling in the pharyngeal area and thus contributes to a balance of resonance from vowel to vowel. Exercise IIIa allows you to slide through these five primary "Italian" vowels.

Now add the following (Exercises VI–X). If any of these exercises are not easy, go back and practice the ones that gave you a sense of release. By no means are these exercises to be tried at one time. Spread them out over several weeks. Master each step as you go along.

EXERCISING YOUR VOICE AND WORKING WITH AIRFLOW

The exercises are impossible to do properly if there is any unrelated force present. The desirable quality at this stage might be compared to tones from an organ being played without the tremolo stop. If the voice begins to wobble around on longer notes, especially on the final one, the production is not correct. Phonation should result from just a thought of pitch and a flow of air with a feeling that everything is loose and open in the throat.

Habits that are established correctly in the first sessions are used as a foundation for all that follows. If they are not established, you have to keep going back to the fundamentals. The more advanced exercises depend on the automatic action of the earlier ones for their free execution.

I place much emphasis on the downward motion in vocalizing. Vocalizing from low to high is encountered almost universally, yet it can be very damaging. The danger lies in a tendency to raise the frequency by increasing the breath pressure. This causes the vocal folds to tighten, which can lead to the formation of vocal nodules and polyps if carried to excess. Prior to studying singing, people's voices have been exercised mostly in the lower third of their range because this is the range of speech. Singing requires the addition of the upper two thirds. Ascending exercises should come later in the training process.

Here are some of the reasons why it is desirable to move from high to low in exercising a voice in early study and in most corrective stages. (This also applies to daily warm-ups.) If you understand that your voice is a wind instrument, the physics of sound dictate that if air pressure is increased, frequency is raised. To convince yourself, try punching your stomach suddenly while sustaining a free tone and see what happens. You have raised the pitch by increasing the subglottal pressure, rather than by letting the vocal folds adjust in response to a thought (Wyke, 1979). We also know that the lungs provide the greatest subglottal pressure when they are full. Thus the singer learns that it is easier to sing at relatively high lung volumes (Proctor, 1979).

If you are trying to find the easiest way to produce tones, it is better not to subject the folds to pressure by pushing. Pressure decreases as the breath goes out. Higher tones require greater pressure (Leanderson & Sundberg, 1988). If we think a pitch, the vocal folds adjust automatically for that frequency without any other force (Leanderson & Sundberg, 1988). The glottis tends to be more relaxed when the respiratory musculature is in an inspiratory rather than an expiratory posture (Minoru Hirano, personal communication, May 15, 1993). In contrast, the vocal folds become more tense as they adjust for higher frequencies (Leanderson & Sundberg, 1988). This tends to match the greater pressure from the lungs when they are filled to start a tone. (The lungs should be comfortably full, not strained to their fullest.) Also, higher pitches should be started lightly because they have more intensity than lower pitches at the same pressure level (see Chapter XV).

Because most of us spend more time speaking than singing, the upper ranges in our voices have had far less exercise than the lower. Therefore, the higher ranges are weaker and need to develop with unstrained exercises over a period of time. The natural inflection of a voice is downward in a sigh or at the end of a sentence. This has been called the "vocal fry." Tone has a natural tendency to move downward as we run out of breath. Curtis (1896) recommends that voices be exercised in downward progressions in their early stages of voice development.

In primitive music, the melody typically progresses downward. (This is a personal observation, and can vary, of course, with the feeling expressed in the music and words.) In primitive and early civilizations, we sang down from the highest tone to the lowest (Thompson, 1939, p. 1622). Today, we build our scales from the bottom up because of the development of harmony based as it is on a fundamental and overtones.

The way the vocal folds are set in motion is the way they will continue to move until a new breath is taken. If the air is expelled with no action of the vocal folds, there is no resistance and, therefore, no sound. If the glottis is closed and expiratory air is pressed against the vocal folds, they are forced apart. Because of the muscle adjustments and the elastic property of the folds, they come together in a cycle of close-open-close-open.

Beginning a sound under these conditions means that the first muscular set of the folds has to be overcome by excessive air pressure. This results in the folds meeting with a slapping action, which can be slight or heavy depending on how tightly the folds were adjusted in the first place. This is known as the "coup de glotte" or "stroke of the glottis." It can be harmful if used habitually and should be avoided in learning to initiate tone. The "fixative" action of the larynx, such as occurs when a person lifts a heavy object, is in this category.

However, if you release a light flow of air and think a sound, the glottis, through which the air is moving, is narrowed, thus reducing pressure to create what is known as the *Bernoulli effect*. Because the energy of the vocal folds is secondary to the energy of the airflow, the subglottal pressure built up by closing the glottis can easily part the folds again, and there is a cycle of open-close-open-close. Initiating a tone in this manner avoids the hyperactivity of the "stroke of the glottis" and allows an easy, free flowing tone production. It is part of the myoelastic-aerodynamic theory of vocal fold vibration. This approach is especially valuable if there has been too much effort in making sound (Van den Berg, 1957). As a part of the whole process, the folds possess a property known as *elastic recoil*, which returns them to their original position (Fink & Demarest, 1978).

LETTING AIRFLOW DO THE WORK

No matter how the above actions are described in writing, the varying combinations will produce different voice qualities. If you imagine that the first airflow is moving at about the same speed as it does when you are making a sound, the flow will be gentle. You can feel the air warm your mouth like steam rising from a boiling kettle. Little air need escape before the tone is started, so that, with the proper kind of silent *h*, it seems as if the tone starts almost immediately. Try to avoid a sudden burst of air. It may take considerable practice to arrive at this point of efficiency, so do not be discouraged if there is excessive air flow at first. The important thing is to **let the air flow do the work**.

For classical singing in the western or European style, the larynx should rest in a low position (Sundberg, 1977). This is sometimes described as being on the brink of a yawn. The larynx should never be pulled down. As explained previously, the larynx will naturally lower a bit by the downward action of the diaphragm in taking a breath. You can feel with your finger the natural lowering of the Adam's apple. Try to develop the sense that the larynx is suspended loosely and see what happens in response to a thought of pitch and a flow of air.

In the Exercises, try to get an inner sense of what your voice can do without listening to it. When you depend on what you hear, it is too late to make an adjustment. The sound has already been made. You are giving attention to what has happened rather than concentrating on what follows. Put cotton in your ears and you will discover what I mean. It takes a great deal of training to trust what comes out if you just let it. Italian soprano Amelita Galli-Curci is reported to have had a studio with very heavy drapes and thick rugs so that she would not depend on those deceptive feedback sounds. Use a tape recorder to find out what you sound like. Another way to sense the voice somewhat as others hear it is to place your hands in front of your ears as you sing, palms facing back, thus principally hearing the sound that is bounced back from the wall.

It will take a number of experiments and a period of time before you can let go sufficiently to be entirely confident that you are allowing phonation to happen. This is the way to start warming up the voice each day.

Great performance is not possible without great technique. Your task is to discover your primal sound and to cultivate it through exercises that release the tone. After a while, it will not take you long to do the warm up exercises. You will develop healthy habits that empower you to give your attention to the words and music.

If you are grappling with the concept of eliciting frequency, I recommend two books: one is *Zen and the Art of Archery* by Eugen Herrigel; the other is *The Inner Game of Tennis* by W. Timothy Gallwey.

If you can learn what it is to float a tone at this stage, the rest is just a matter of patience and time. *Think* what you want and *let* it happen. Then *trust* the result.

REFERENCES

Curtis, H.H. (1973). *Voice building and tone placement*, Minneapolis, Mn: Pro-Musica Press. (Reprinted 1909, New York: D. Appleton, 3rd Ed.) (original published 1896).

Fink, B., & Demarest, R.J. (1978). *Laryngeal biomechanics*, Cambridge, Ma: Harvard University Press, p. 65.

Leanderson, R., & Sundberg, J. (1988). *Breathing for singing*, in Journal of Voice, Vol. 2, #1, New York: Raven Press, p. 2.

Merriam-Webster's eighth new collegiate dictionary (1981). Springfield, Ma: Merriam-Webster.

Proctor, D.F. (1979). *Breath, the power source of the voice*, Transcripts of the 8th Symposium, Care of the professional voice, Part II, New York: The Voice Foundation, p. 14.

Sundberg, J. (1974). *Acoustic interpretation of the singer's formant*, Journal of the Acoustical Society of America, 55, p. 838–844.

Sundberg, J. (1977, March). *The acoustics of the singing voice,* Scientific American, p. 82.

Thompson, O. (1939). *International Cyclopedia of Music & Musicians,* New York: Mead, p. 1622.

Van den Berg, J. (1957). *On the air resistance and the Bernoulli effect of the human larynx,* Journal of the Acoustical Society of America, #29, p. 626–631.

Wyke, B. (1979). *Neurological aspects of phonatory control systems in the larynx,* in Transcripts of the 8th Symposium, care of the professional voice, Part II, New York: The Voice Foundation, p. 42.

V

■

RANGE AND REGISTERS

Emme Calve (1858–1942) was especially famous for her interpretation of Carmen, yet she also enjoyed great acclaim for her coloratura roles of Lucia, Lakme and Ophelia. Her range extended from F above high C down to A below the staff. Joan Sutherland started as a mezzo and then became the great coloratura soprano we can hear on records. Marilyn Horne was first a lyric soprano, then the phenomenal mezzo-soprano we all admire. Lauritz Melchior and James King both were baritones before they found their heldentenor voices. On the other hand, Leonard Warren experimented with tenor before becoming a dramatic baritone. Many more singers could be named who have exceptional ranges or who changed classification as their voices developed.

As young children, many of us have ranges of over three octaves. I said this at my first voice seminar in 1972 and one of the teachers who had come with his family taped the voice of his two-year-old boy while playing with him. I have a copy of this tape, which demonstrates a range of sounds from D6, which is a ninth above high C down to B2, which is the second line of the bass clef.

Voices have a much greater potential range than most students realize. I have had students who could vocalize above the top notes of the piano and others practically off the lower end. I question the usefulness of these extreme ranges, but voices can do it. There have been exceptional singers who exceeded three octaves in performance—Yma Sumac and Ivan Rebroff, for example. What does this mean to you as a student? It means that you should explore your potential before you accept a label.

THE VOICE AS MUSICAL INSTRUMENT

With the exception of early Greek drama, where it seems that actors used exceptionally wide ranges (Daitz, 1978), early music frequently consisted of entire melodies written within an octave or a tenth. Look up ancient tunes, plainsong, folk music or the earliest operatic scores, and you will find that vocalists were seldom expected to reach excessively high or low notes. Beginning in the seventeenth and eighteenth centuries, however, operatic composers seeking to convey a wider range of emotional expression began to think of the voice as a musical instrument. Handel and Haydn demanded great technical facility, while Mozart, Weber, and Donizetti further extended vocal range and dynamics.

Today, we find composers using considerable vocal range and vocalists exploring a variety of qualities as well (some, to a degree that jeopardizes their vocal health). Vocal range takes many years to develop, and no singer can know how much range he has until he experiments. At first, it will seem to the novice that she has several different voices because of the different qualities between her high, middle, and low notes. This diversity is natural. Similar changes can also be found in other musical instruments. For example, the high notes of the clarinet do not sound like the low. This is also true of the French horn, violin, oboe—in fact, all musical instruments.

UNDERSTANDING YOUR VOCAL RANGE

The contrasting qualities in vocal range are referred to as registers, which Webster's (Merriam-Webster, 1981) defines as "a musical range or compass, or a particular portion of the compass on an instrument or voice, of which all the tones are produced in the same manner or are similar in quality."

The wide discrepancy of opinion as to how many registers there are stems from the kind of understanding one has of how the various parts of the voice function. I'm reminded of a student who had previously studied with a coloratura soprano, so she could sing coloratura. Later, she studied with a mezzo so she could sing mezzo. Still later, she studied with a dramatic soprano, so she could sing dramatic music. After she had worked with me on technique for about two months, I gave her a piece of music to learn. The first day we tried it she stopped the accompanist and asked, "Which voice do you want me to use?" She had not yet learned that she had a mezzo voice of considerable size, with good range and agility as a whole, not divided into parts.

As you seek to discover your own vocal range, remember that each voice has range, size, and agility of its own. And since each student has his or her own "voice print," he or she will have his own particular vocal quality as well. A voice is a voice. Each has the same fundamental anatomy and physiology as all other voices. Yet each has characteristics that make it unique. As students and teachers of singing, we must learn what adjustments are possible and how they can be coordinated.

SOME DEFINITIONS OF REGISTER

Many terms have been used to identify the various qualities that are heard in different parts of the range. *High* and *low pitches* have been called *light* and *heavy, thin* and *thick, falsetto* and *chest* or, often *head, middle,* and *chest.* Other English terms have been used, along with the foreign language names for the same qualities. Unfortunately, voice scientists, doctors, and voice teachers have developed separate vocabularies, which compound the difficulty of explaining exactly what happens in these so-called registers.

In 1983, Harry Hollein presented "A View of Vocal Registers" at the 12th Symposium on Care of the Professional Voice, sponsored by the Voice Foundation. The report was based on the outcome of a study on vocal registers by a committee that included physicians, scientists, and voice pedagogues. Giving each register a number, starting with the lowest, they defined the registers as follows:

Register 1: The very lowest of registers, probably used only in speaking (old terms: *pulse, vocal fry, creak*).

Register 2: That (low) register, which is used by most for speaking and singing (old terms: *modal, chest, normal* and *heavy*).

Register 3: A high register used primarily in singing (old terms: *falsetto, light, head*).

Register 4: A very high register found in some women and children and particularly relevant to the coloratura soprano (old terms: *flute, whistle*).

At the same symposium, we referred to yet another register, 2A, which stood for that register in the middle of the frequency range that constitutes a problem in training many singers. (Old terms for register 2A would include *head, mid, middle,* and *upper.*)

An alternative approach would be to use as labels a pair of terms such as *heavy/light,* or a second set, *lower/upper.* (A thorough reading of this report is valuable for those interested in learning more about how the committee reached their conclusions.)

Think for a moment about the different registers you hear outside of classical singing. In Switzerland, a yodel is traditional. Similar sounds are heard in country-western singing in the United States and in Hispanic folk songs of Latin America. Tibetans use a yodel when calling to a distance and African pygmies use the same mechanism when singing. The cowboy and "hog caller" use the falsetto "break." These sounds are used by both males and females with great gusto.

REGISTER ADJUSTMENT

So what is meant by *register adjustment?* It means that you learn to bridge over one register into the range of another and add the second register without letting go of the first. It is a coordination or integration of all parts of the range so that there is a smooth transition between high and low. A film called *The Falsetto Voice,* by Henry Rubin and Charles Hirt, illustrates this beautifully.

In the following discussion, bear in mind that there can be considerable variety from one voice to another. The upper notes of Register 2 for a tenor would be higher than Register 2 for a baritone, and Register 2 for a baritone would be higher than Register 2 for a bass. The same would apply to women's voices for the upper part of Register 2—soprano higher than mezzo, and so on (Figure V–1).

John McCormick was criticized for using falsetto in his soft, high singing because many critics did not understand voice well enough to recognize that, in his lyric voice, he had very beautifully integrated the falsetto with chest, upper with lower. Richard Tucker was a master, as was Leo Slezak, at passing from forte to pianissimo in any range of the voice. The upper and lower limits or "shift points" of all registers must be evaluated on an individual basis. To understand what causes problems in registration, it is necessary to know the student's history—to know what concept has been used in guiding the voice so far. Bear in mind that the voice responds to mental concepts.

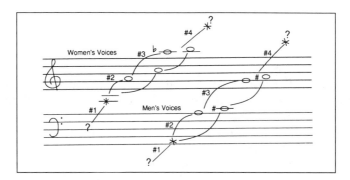

Figure V–1. Approximate ranges of registers #1—#2—#3—#4. The * indicates the upper and lower limits of voice range—a variable with each voice. The slur marks indicate limits of range within each register; the slur above represents a higher voice, and the slur underneath represents a lower voice.

After puberty, the untrained Register 2 voice—the part of the range used in every day conversation by both males and females—has, on average, a natural upward extension to about middle C for the male voice, and an octave higher, third space C for the female voice. For a bass voice, the changing point can be B or Bb, and for a lyric tenor, a C-sharp. Correspondingly, for a mezzo or alto, the limit can be third line B or B-flat; while for a coloratura soprano, it can be C-sharp. This observation has been borne out a number of times by students who had "perfect pitch." They would confess that they had difficulty in knowing "which way" to sing at these particular pitches. The terminology *which way* is significant because it indicates the student has realized that a different kind of "adjustment" takes place at these points. A young male will sing up the scale and, if he is not pushing, say that he can't go higher than middle C (for example) unless he changes to falsetto.

EXPLORING REGISTERS OF YOUR VOICE

In exploring the various registers of the voice, I start with Register 2 or the "speaking voice," because that is the part the student knows best. The exercises in the previous chapter have already started us in this direction. You should have started eliciting pitch before proceeding in this chapter. Review Exercises I through X in the appendix and as explained in Chapter IV, if necessary.

DISCUSSION: REGISTERS 2 AND 3

Register 2 uses the thyroarytenoid muscles without activation of the cricothyroides in the untrained voice. (Remember that the vocal folds and the thyroarytenoids are the same thing.) Even in this limited segment of the range, the upper part is seldom used in everyday conversation.

Register 2 is strong because you have used it all your life. Register 3 employs an additional pair of muscles, the cricothyroids. When the cricothyroid muscles are activated they put a longitudinal force on the vocal folds, making the folds longer and thinner. One hundred years ago, Holbrook Curtis (1896) wrote that if a singer has lost the use of the cricothyroid muscles, he is no longer able to produce high tones. If the thyroarytenoids are relaxed, the result will be a light, breathy quality—the falsetto. In this action, the vocal folds do not meet at the midline.

If the thyroarytenoids are activated at the same time, as they are elongated by the cricothyroids, they tend to thicken and therefore fill the gap. It is by learning how to keep the cricothyroids active at the same time that the thyroarytenoids are added that you start to exercise the mixed voice (or *voix-mixe* as the French call it). It is an antagonistic action. Eventually you learn to carry Register 3 (falsetto) almost to the bottom of your range and the Register 2 (chest) almost to the top. This should be done with the larynx resting in a low position. It is impossible later to develop the operatic or classical tone if the larynx is raised. Register 2 should be carried up very lightly. If you have not exercised the #3 register from the beginning of your study, it can take a very long time.

A low larynx position can be induced by the feeling of a beginning yawn—no pulling down! The position can also be gained with the sensation of a raised soft palate, which induces the larynx to lower reflexively.

I like to use the following diagram to illustrate the interplay between the two principle registers: falsetto (Register 3) and chest (Register 2) (Figure V–2): The whole represents the integrated voice, from top to bottom. If the full, even range of the voice were represented by the outside lines, there would be a mixture of light to the bottom of the range and heavy to the top of the range in varying proportions of muscular input. In soft, high singing there would be less activation of Register 2 adjustment and in loud singing, more. Throughout the range, the proportion of light and heavy is constantly changing. I realize that this illustration is idealized, but I haven't found a better way to represent what we are striving for.

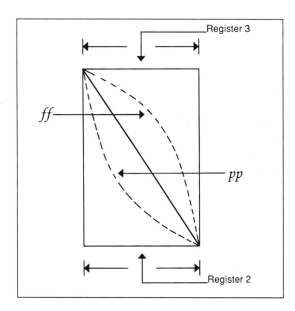

Figure V–2. Interplay between two principle registers.

REGISTER 3

To discover Register 3, think a light, childish tone at about A, A-flat or G above the staff (an octave lower for the male voice). Take an easy breath and release a gentle flow of air, sighing a soft *Huh* [hə], and let it slide in a downward inflection, without definite pitches (Exercise XI). I ask female students to think of a little girl sound and male students to think of a woman's voice. As the air flows through the glottis, its action on the covering mucosa will draw the vocal folds together in vibration.

Some students find it easier to blow gently with rounded lips, like cooling a hot drink and then release a soft "Hoo" [hu]. This vowel helps because rounded lips induce the reflex action of sucking, which tends to lower the larynx.

Occasionally, students are more successful with a light *m* hum. Use the same gentle downward inflection, without trying to "sing" it: "Hmmmmmmmm." Remember that an *m* hum is like *uh* with the lips closed, tongue passive. It is rare that a student will find this new quality by starting from a lower tone. Letting the voice become lighter and almost breathy as it slides up is possible and desirable later on.

The problems involved in exercising Register 3 can be psychological. The derivation of the word *falsetto* goes back to the past participle of the Latin verb *falere*, to deceive. To the extent that we associate falsetto with something *false* or *wrong*, we may have built a mental barrier against it. Also, it is unfortunate that so many claim that there is no such thing in the female voice. Physiological findings are identical in the female voice to those in the male voice, only an octave higher. I remember reading an interview with Dorothy Kirsten in the *New York Times* (commemorating her 30th year at the Metropolitan Opera) in which she stated that in her early training, she studied with an old German teacher who made her practice with her "falsetto voice" for a full year (*New York Times*, 12/20/1975).

Male singers may be hesitant to use Register 3 at first because it is so unfamiliar to them. Many female singers do not recognize this area in their voices because their voices change so little at puberty. They have been accustomed to the light, high quality all their lives. Others, however, have to discover this part of the voice, especially those who have been singing popular music, using only the lower range.

When the new Register 3 (falsetto) quality is discovered, think a definite pitch and slide it down an octave. (Exercises XII and XIIA) This is called *portamento*. Repeat a half step lower, following a descending sequence. Start each top note with the same "new" Register 3 quality as in the preceding exercise. Learn to carry this light adjustment down through A or A-flat middle range or lower.

Once a smooth connection has been found, the voice should be exercised in this manner from two to five minutes at each practice session. Do not try to use this new voice in song in the beginning stages. In time, you will achieve a sensation that all notes are being produced in the same spot, and that there is an even flow of air from note to note.

A "break" occurs when the light, upper mechanism reaches the lower, heavier mechanism and suddenly lets go. At that point, feel a sense of yawning space at the back of your throat and let the tones be even lighter and more breathy. This helps to bridge over the gap with no perceptible break. Some singers can do this in the first lesson, while others may have to work at it for several weeks. Blending Registers 3 and 2 is the foundation of the "seamless scale." Tenors need to exercise the lower part of the Register 3 voice in order to manage the D to A range above middle C. Basses and baritones, especially, must let the voice lighten and loosen above middle C.

Some years ago, a young baritone found his Register 3 voice and began to show in his lessons that he understood how to make a smooth connection into Register 2. Because he could do this, I was greatly puzzled when, after a few weeks, he had difficulty singing the falsetto notes as freely as when he'd begun. I asked him what he was doing in his own practice. He said he thought it was just the same as in the studio. Quite by chance the following week I overheard him practicing in the morning, again in the afternoon, and again in the evening. He must have worked nearly an hour each time—and practically all falsetto! I called him in the next day to find out how long he had been doing this. He replied he had done it ever since he had found out how. I asked why he practiced it so long each day, and he said he thought that would strengthen the muscle faster. By dropping back the falsetto practice to no more than three to six minutes, two or three times a day, his voice began to behave and his tones to strengthen.

If you can slide from Register 3 into Register 2 without a break, you are ready to add Exercises XIII and XIV. The portamento from bottom to top should take you back to the same light quality you started with. It is necessary to lighten the voice immediately when ascending. No weight of quality from a lower note should be carried into the next higher note. You are sensitizing your ears and the feelings of the muscles in your throat to a new but natural part of the voice.

The female often has more difficulty finding her low voice than the male. And yet, most females speak in the Register 2 range. They have not learned to associate a prolongation of sound and a definite pitch with this speaking quality. When practiced by starting below middle C and exercising gently upward through the middle range, this register can go much higher than supposed. The chest voice should not be used exclusively as many popular singers do. As you get to second line G and above, your voice should get looser and lighter to blend with Register 3. For low notes, Jennie Tourel always asked her students to relax the voice into a speaking quality.

Lilli Lehman (1909) had these things to say on the subject: "The head voice [#3] is the most valuable possession of all singers, male and female. Without its aid all voices lack brilliancy and carrying power. It is absolutely necessary for the artist to give consideration to his falsetto . . . . I must form the lowest notes in such a way that I can reach the highest. In descending, I must preserve very carefully the form taken for the highest tone . . . .

must think it higher, never lower . . . . I imagine I am striking the same tone again. In singing a high tone I feel the energy of the tension increases from head to foot, a stretching lengthwise . . . . With every tone, the singer must feel he can go higher" (Excerpts from "How to Sing").

REGISTER 1

To find the lowest notes in Register 1, the larynx must rest in a very relaxed, low position and then apply an almost breathy flow of air. It takes more air flow and less pressure to produce low notes than high ones because the vocal folds are looser (that is, they do not come together so often) and the amount of air that escapes at each open phase is greater. Any attempt to produce these notes by tensing and pushing down into them prevents the muscles from performing their natural function and shuts off the resonance. For this part of the voice, let the tone slide down and let the air flow do the work (Exercise XV).

In Register 1, the thyroarytenoids are considerably shortened and thickened. I hypothesize that the external thyoarytenoid muscle is somehow involved in producing the lowest notes of the bass register. In my own voice, I can feel a distinct muscle activity taking place at about A to G, bottom of the bass clef. I hear the same thing happening in the lowest women's voices, one octave higher, A to G below middle C. I find practically nothing written about the exact range in which Register 1 becomes a part of the low notes for a singer. I feel sure that the external thyroarytenoid muscles contribute to the strength or intensity of the lowest notes of a low voice. (See Figure XVI–2 in Chapter XVI.)

REGISTER 4

For those who are able, discovering Register 4 (flute) is very much the same as finding Register 3. It should be started perhaps at B, C, or D above the staff (for the male voice, an octave lower). A humming sound or the smallest kind of lip opening in a position for "oo" [u] can be tried with absolutely no tensing of the lips, jaw, or throat, and with a gentle flow of air. (No reaching for the note!)

When it is first discovered, it seems to pop out from nowhere. It just happens. It may not always be on the pitch you were think-ing. Most likely, you will have a distinct feeling that you had nothing to do with creating the sound and that you had no control over it. It will seem like an entirely different voice. If the note doesn't pop out by itself, forget it. Never try to "make" it. Never push (Exercise XVI).

Another exercise to discover Register 4 is to use a very light staccato in an arpeggio (Exercise XVII). The top note should be the lightest. I can't tell you how many students have said, after discovering this part of the voice, "I used to make sounds like that before I studied." That is exactly what my first student told me after some months of loosening her jaw and throat. She was petite. When she first came to me, the veins would stand out on her neck and she would get very red in the face on any notes at the top of the staff. Her teachers had told her she was a dramatic soprano and she was trying to prove it. We found she was a light coloratura.

These light, high tones should only be practiced a few minutes at a time at first. Just play with them. Don't expect any real application of these high notes for several months or even years. This is the part of the voice used by every coloratura for her highest pitches. Listen to the recordings of Frieda Hemple, Amelita Galli-Curci, Joan Sutherland, and other great artists. These women practiced for years before they produced the finished product that you hear.

In all of these exercises, the jaw must hang loosely with the tongue either resting behind the lower teeth or out on the lower lip. Your mouth does not need to open widely for either high or low notes. I sometimes call the position a "dumb jaw." Cheek muscles are loose with no tensing or drawing back of the corners of the mouth. Do not push to extend your range in any direction. Good, open space is needed inside the mouth, in the pharyngeal area.

The flute voice, Register 4, is more characteristic of the female than the male, although some males can find it quite easily. Scientific investigation is not conclusive about what action takes place, but there is a hypothesis that a "damping" action produces these highest notes. It begins to take over at B-flat or B above the staff and extends upward. No extra pushing is required to discover this Register. In fact, quite the opposite is needed. The throat muscles must be very relaxed and only the lightest kind of airflow may be used to produce what seems to be a very breathy, weak sound. If you try to find these highest pitches by straining to raise Register 3 higher, you are doomed to failure.

Flute voice is not only of value to the coloratura. Listen, for example, to Leontyne Price and hear the easy approach she has to her top notes. She is not a coloratura, but it is because she has practiced notes higher than she sings publicly that she can do what she does. In other words, she is not reaching for the upper limits of her range, but has room to spare. Birgit Nilsson used the *Queen of the Night* aria's to vocalize. Also, listen to the old time bass, Pol Plancon, for light, upper voice use. The better we can sensitize and exercise all the fine muscle fibers that lie within the vocal folds, the better control we have for high notes, soft notes, full notes, flexibility, and all the gradations in between.

EXERCISING YOUR VOICE—THE RIGHT WAY

It is important to exercise the voice every day. When regularly called upon, the rested nerves become more sensitive and responsive. Perhaps you have rested an arm, wrist, or some other part of your body because of a strain and noticed when you started using it again, that it was very weak. This is exactly what happens when you don't exercise your voice. Of course, if you are physically tired, a day of no singing might be a good thing. Likewise, a day of very little use after several days of regular or intense use is advisable.

Exercises starting from the bottom can be practiced with a light staccato. The upper notes should adjust automatically with just the thought of the pitches. They may feel very detached at first. This not only leads to the "seamless scale," but is also a foundation for coloratura later on (Exercises XVII & XVIIA).

Another way to think when trying to achieve a blend is to imagine that we begin to lighten the Register 2 voice gradually when going higher and again lighten the Register 3 voice gradually when going lower. Another approach is to feel the Register 3 voice take over as you go higher and the Register 2 voice take over as you go lower, both parts continuing to function with varying intensities simultaneously.

Throughout the range, the proportion of light to heavy is constantly changing. The proportion of Register 3 is greater above approximately middle C for the male, and above the B or C an octave higher for the female (depending on voice classification, higher for high voices, lower for low voices). Ideally, both the light and heavy are working all the time. There is a greater proportion of light in a lyric voice and a greater proportion of heavy in a dramatic voice.

The ideal is a "one register" system. The "two register" adherents would probably recognize the different adjustments of lower and upper, but would not admit to the possibility of their integration. The "three register" adherents would go part way in this training, getting a mixture in the middle of the range but then letting go of the upper when the voice began to get too low and, inversely, letting go of the lower when the voice began to get too high. In the female voice this is manifest in the so-called "passagio" around E–F above middle C and again an octave higher. The same thing takes place in the male voice, especially around E, F, and G above middle C for the tenor voice. I believe this is because too heavy a lower adjustment has been carried too high and the upper has not had the opportunity to strengthen its lower extension. Pitch problems often arise from improper muscular adjustments rather than wrong hearing. Think of the passagio as near "C" in both voices: middle C, men; third space C, women.

This study should be done with the guidance of an experienced teacher who understands the physiology of vocal production and has a well-trained ear to help identify the right kind of sound. The human voice is capable of so many variations; the ear must be trained to differentiate sounds that are healthy and can lead to good, integrated action from sounds that are limiting or downright harmful if repeated in exercises. A rule of thumb: if it is not comfortable, it is probably harmful. At this point of development, an aesthetically beautiful sound is not necessarily the criterion. That comes in time with the right kind of exercise practiced for the right amount of time. Just a short period of practice is best at first for these new muscle adjustments. Remember the basic rule for singing, that it is better to do too little than to do too much.

All parts of the voice need to be exercised. A typical illustration of the singer who does not exercise the loft voice, Register 3, for example, is the church soloist who has rehearsals perhaps twice a week during the winter season, but does not sing much during the summer. As this singer reaches her late thirties or early forties (I have noticed it particularly in females), the voice begins to develop a wobble and to lose its high notes. I have worked with many such singers and rehabilitated their voices by reactivating the Register 3 mechanism with light exercises from the top down. Some singers who come to me have not performed for 20 to 25 years. Through practice, they rediscover their voices sufficiently to sing church solos and give recitals—and be asked back!

Sometimes the reverse occurs, however. I remember a young man who began lessons with me singing tenor in a light, almost falsetto voice and discovered that he was really a bass. A 38-year-old soprano came to me singing in her unchanged "little girl" voice, only to discover she was actually a mezzo. Both of these singers have maintained their new voices over a period of years and enjoyed local professional success.

By repeating this voyage of discovery a little bit each day, you will gradually achieve better control. As your voice produces notes more easily at one end of the range, the notes at the other end also become easier. I believe this is due to the fact that the throat muscles must be free of all forcing for both high and low adjustments.

The fundamental principles for extending range and blending registers has been stated above. There will be exceptions, of course. Perhaps not enough of the preliminary exercises described in Chapter IV were mastered to bring about conditions permitting an extension of range and blending of registers. There may be anatomical differences in the size of the various muscle bundles that limit the potential for developing certain parts of the voice. We are not all equally endowed.

A singer is a vocal athlete who must keep his or her laryngeal muscles in condition through regular exercise. This goes for both professionals and amateurs who wish to maintain good vocal health. I hasten to add that the correct kind of vocalizing must be used, of course. This point was charmingly illustrated by a student who exhibited considerable difficulty in his first lesson with me. When I asked him about his previous study, he explained that he had worked with an opera singer who retired at the age of 19! Any questions?

Technique is the process of knowing what to do and how to do it. Happily, it is also the easiest way to do a piece of work. Develop your voice stage by stage, or you will find yourself in trouble. It is much harder to unlearn faulty habits than to practice good ones. As Maria Callas said, "If you start right, you are right for life. But if you start wrong, it's hard later to correct bad habits" (Ardoin, 1987, p. 3).

It takes much discipline to be successful in voice study. There are no short-cuts. You will be richly rewarded if you are not in too much of a hurry. There is great satisfaction in feeling good about your singing as you gradually uncover new sensations and add new notes to your range. By degrees, you will begin to feel that singing is a natural part of you, that it is a means of expressing your inner feelings. When singing is approached in a healthy manner, your throat will feel good after each practice. You should always stop while your throat is feeling good. Do not fatigue your voice by singing too long. Each day, start from the beginning and warm up. You can't expect a "cold" voice to sound the way it did when you finished exercising it the day before.

By the process of *thinking* of what you have to work with and why it works that way, you can commence the routine of *letting* it happen. Then *trust* the result.

REFERENCES

Ardoin, J. (1987). *Callas at Juilliard*, New York: Knopf (p. 3).

Curtis, H.H. (1973). *Voice building and tone placement*, Minneapolis, Mn: Pro-Musica Press. (Reprinted 1909, New York: D. Appleton, 3rd ed.) (Original published 1896.)

Daitz, S., (1978). *A recital of Ancient Greek Poetry*, New York: Norton.

Hollein, H., (1983). *A report on vocal registers*. Care of the professional voice, Part I, New York: The Voice Foundation, (p. 5).

Lehman, L., (1909). *How to sing* (R. Aldrich, Trans.). New York: Macmillan.

Merriam-Webster. *Eighth new collegiate dictionary.* (1981). Springfield, Ma: Merriam-Webster.

The New York Times. (1975). *Dorothy Kirsten.* (From group interview, December 30.)

VI

■

VOICE CLASSIFICATION: CHILDREN'S VOICES

Having explored range and register, you might wonder what kind of voice you are: soprano or mezzo, baritone or tenor? You might mull over the subdivisions, such as spinto, lyric, coloratura, dramatic, bass-baritone, heldentenor, and all the rest which reflect the influence of opera on the history of voice use. To this I say, "First of all, you are a *voice*!"

What elements of a voice lead to a specific label? Size, range, color, flexibility, character, length of time you can sing before getting tired, and the technique used to integrate a smooth transition between high and low or soft and loud. To know your *tessitura* is most important. It is the range between the top and bottom notes of your voice where you can perform most comfortably for the longest period of time without fatigue.

You were born with some qualities that cannot be acquired in any other way. Others may be gained by technical development. If you have a big voice, you must learn to sing softly. If you do not have a big voice, nothing can make it big except to have it amplified by a microphone. Size is not everything, however, nor is it the most important attribute. Many light voices have an excellent carrying quality, Kathleen Battle being the preeminent example among classical singers today.

BE WARY OF CLASSIFICATION

Classification is a tricky business. It would be a great injustice to restrict singers to any special voice type before they have had time to explore their range and dynamics and to develop their technique. As you know, to acquire technique is to learn what to do and how to do it in the easiest possible manner. Since every voice student is different, there are no hard and fast rules. Add to this the fact that individuals mature at different rates and you can appreciate how complicated classification can be. I urge young singers to be on their guard against the "fach" system, which is the custom in so many of the German opera houses. To limit a young talent in this manner can inhibit growth. It can also restrict the range and color of the voice to the point of being harmful. Artists beware: most house managers are only interested in having their immediate needs satisfied.

Let me tell you about two mezzos who came to me within a month of each other. Both were in their late twenties and had sung mezzo through high school and college. As we vocalized, we discovered that both singers had high ranges they had never explored. As teenagers, their choral directors had placed them in the alto section because they could read music, and so they had become mezzos. After some period of study, a production of Mozart's *Impresario* was given with these singers doing the coloratura parts. They have since been very comfortable with their "new" voices.

I am reminded of another student whose first teacher trained her as a mezzo. Her second teacher found that she could not carry this low quality up, but discovered that she had some high notes and, therefore, declared her a soprano. Some years later, she came to me with the problem of a big break in her voice between high and low. By learning how to bridge this break, we discovered that her best range was her lower voice, and that she could connect this smoothly with the upper notes—the overall tessitura being mezzo.

Another case was that of a lyric baritone who was particularly good at singing high, soft notes. He had the opportunity to be presented in a New York Town Hall Recital which was reviewed by critics from both *The New York Times* and *The Herald Tribune*. Both critics made note of his fine high notes and predicted that he would one day be a tenor. After this performance, a year went by before this young man came to me for further study. I was surprised to find that he was having great difficulty with his top voice. During the year he had been on his own, he had sung tenor in his church choir because of what the critics wrote. Through careful work, we were able to restore his natural, lyric baritone, but it took nearly a year to do so.

I know of no shortcuts in determining a classification. In my experience, attempting one produces only a short-cut to the end of any thoughts of a career.

A good teacher or a vocal coach who thoroughly understands healthy voice use is probably the safest guide in your search for a particular voice classification. This is especially true because you have only a vague idea of how you sound to others. Of course, you may have a preference, but that is not a safe criterion for establishing your classification.

In the following chapters there are exercises for further technical development of the voice. Don't be in a hurry to limit yourself in classification. Claudia Muzio was known as the singer with three voices: lyric, dramatic, and coloratura. Many singers start out in one category and then change to another as they mature. Flagstad was lyric before becoming a Wagnerian soprano. She also had excellent coloratura facility, including a perfect trill, in her technique.

WORKING WITH CHILDREN'S VOICES

At this point in discovering a voice, a few comments about children's voices might be appropriate. In unchanged children's voices there is very little difference anatomically or physiologically between male and female. At puberty, the male larynx grows larger and the voice range drops approximately an octave. The female voice can change to as much as a third lower in range, but it is the overall "maturity" of the sound which impresses.

The principles described in Chapters IV and V apply to young voices as well, although you cannot expect full, mature sounds from children, who have not yet finished growing. The average human has not completed his physical development until age 21.

Young voices need to practice lightly over a period of time before changes take place. I know of those who put on operas with unchanged and teenage voices. Once when I questioned a teacher about this practice, she replied, "These students may never get a chance to perform in opera if they don't do it now!" On the contrary, I suspect that if young voices perform opera while they are still in their teens, they will never get the chance to perform when they are older. Adelina Patti, Ernestine Schumann-Heink, and Conchita Supervia are the exceptions, not the rule, all of them having started professional singing before they were seventeen. This is not even a handful out of thousands of students in a period of less than a hundred years. And although Patti gave concerts as a child prodigy between the ages of seven and twelve, she had a period of rest before making her operatic debut at sixteen. Patti's recordings were made when she was in her sixties.

Children should not be required to sing in any but their light voices. A boy might sing in his alto voice and then become a tenor, as Jussi Bjorling did. It was Bjorling's good fortune to be in the hands of his father, who knew what was healthy for his voice. More often than not, young boys who sing in children's choirs are asked to sing like a mature female soprano and, if they are good, are kept in their solo positions far too long. I have known of many such cases, where boys lost interest in singing after their voices changed—especially since they had great difficulty relating their "changed" voices to singing.

The histories of damage done to young voices in Broadway shows such as *Annie* are notorious. High school productions of Broadway musicals have also left a trail of strained and abused talent. With careful guidance it is possible to put on these shows, but the students should not be required to practice too long at a time and should be cautioned not to imitate the Broadway professionals, many of whom have trouble maintaining healthy voice use themselves.

As Joel J. Pressman wrote many years ago, "The force of the expiratory blast of the lungs of a growing child is ordinarily greater in proportion than the state of development of the vocal cords; so forceful, prolonged use is proportionately greater trauma to the vocal cords. There is no better way to ruin a promising career than too early and too enthusiastic training" (1940, p. 281).

A young person was referred to me with vocal nodules. She had been studying singing for fifteen years, but she was only eighteen years old! The nodules disappeared after a short time with voice therapy treatment but I do not have a follow-up to report because her home was over 500 miles from St. Louis, where she had been referred for treatment. This is a clear illustration, however, of what happens when too much is done too soon.

In my own experience, there is no damage done to the young male's voice if he is allowed to sing lightly during the voice change at puberty. There should definitely be no forcing. One junior high voice teacher had great success by having her male students sing only those notes that were written within easy range. When tones were too high or too low, the students just followed the music silently and then came in again when the notes were within easy reach. I have worked with male students during their puberty, and sang myself during that time, sometimes baritone and sometimes soprano. Fortunately, I was never required to sing for long periods.

WHAT IS A MONOTONE?

The question of "monotones" is frequently raised. My answer is that there is no such thing. Medically, if you find a true monotone, it is reported that he will be dead in three minutes. I compare the monotone question to the problem some people have with vision. There are those who can match a color they see today one month later. Others are insensitive to color and could not match two samples exactly if their lives depended on it. Yet, they could see a difference between blue and yellow, for example. Sensitivity to pitch is similarly varied.

While some children are known to have perfect pitch at age three, others do not make fine distinctions until they are much older. I once remarked to a group of college students studying to be teachers that there is no such thing as a monotone. From the back of the room I heard one of them exclaim, " Oh yeah?" I invited that young lady to speak with me after class. She told me that in the first grade her teacher told her that she was a monotone, so she never sang. Because she liked music, she had learned to play the piano. Experimenting with different sounds she could make, we found she had nearly a three-octave range. I agreed to teach her, and in three months she was singing low voice in a girls trio. She subsequently went back to school to study music and later got a position teaching music in the public schools.

One way to help those who lack sensitivity to pitch is to match their sounds to notes on the piano. For example, I might ask a student to sustain a single word such as "I." Then, by finding the corresponding note on the piano, the student could begin the process of relating what he heard with his ears with what he was doing with his voice. Games of imitating a fire siren or other sounds can also bring about an awareness of the difference between high and low tones. A cry of joy can be contrasted with a moan of pain—in both cases relating the sounds to pitches on the piano. It is a slow process, but I have found that progress can be made.

PRESERVING CHILDREN'S VOICES

I want to repeat that, in training children's voices, no attempt should be made to have them sing loudly or for too long at one time. Singing should be fun. It should be a happy experience of discovering different parts of the voice. The pressure placed on children to achieve goals beyond their years very often comes from ambitious parents. In that case, the parents should be invited to attend the lessons and learn what a child's voice is capable of doing.

I once attended an audition of children's voices for a radio program. One little girl sang with a pushed and squeezed quality that sounded like no one else. The director of the program immediately gave special attention because her voice was so distinctive. When I spoke to him about the danger to her vocal health because of the way she was singing, he replied that he didn't care about that because the quality would get attention on his program. He said that if her voice gave out, he would find someone else.

In working with children's voices, the teacher or director must do a great deal of *thinking* for the child. If he or she can help the child to learn how to *let* natural sounds come out without pushing or trying to imitate another's quality, a foundation will be established which will give the child confidence to *trust* the result.

REFERENCES

Pressman, J.J. (1940). *Physiology of the larnyx—A resume and discussion for the literature for 1939. Laryngoscope, 50,* (#4) p. 281.

VII

■

AGILITY

Have you ever thought of being a ballet dancer or a tightrope artist? Perhaps you dreamed of being a diver or a figure skating champion? Can you imagine diving from a high board and entering the water with hardly a splash the first time? It takes months and years of practice to realize such feats. Martha Graham (1991) has said that "it takes about ten years to make a mature dancer" (p. 4). And yet I have known young students of singing who thought they could audition for opera before they had learned to sing fast runs and skips, a skill that is known as *agility*.

I have referred to singers as vocal athletes, but what sets them apart from other athletes is the location and nature of muscles involved in vocal production. The muscles of the larynx are minuscule compared to the muscles dancers and divers use, and we cannot see or feel with our fingers what is taking place when we make a sound. Yet, there is a parallel: Singers must train like all athletes to establish kinesthetic responses.

Many of us have all witnessed dazzling exhibitions of coloratura carried out with a daring that borders on the super-human. It adds excitement to a performance equal to that of any high wire act at a circus. More important, however, is what this skill does for the singer. I agree with Jerome Hines, who told me that he feels that flexibility is the lifeline of the voice.

THE VALUE OF LEARNING COLORATURA

In the days of "bel canto," it was standard for all students to learn coloratura. Listen to the recordings of Luisa Tetrazzini, Ernestine Schumann-Heink, Ferrando DeLucia, and Pol Plancon, to name a soprano, contralto, tenor and bass, and you will hear what the training produced. More recently, we have Joan Sutherland, Marylin Horne, Richard Tucker, and Samuel Ramey as examples. In addition, there must be a significant correlation between having this skill and having a long career. Jerome Hines has been singing for over forty years. I was privileged to hear both Tetrazzini and Schumann-Heink in their sixties and can bear witness to the remarkable freshness of their voices as well as their ability to execute coloratura.

Remember that coloratura refers to ornamental passages, runs and embellishments, not just to a high soprano voice. The male singer is just as capable of fast runs, skips, and trills as the female. As a basis for healthy technique, it is just as valuable today as it ever was. What can have happened to the human voice in 150 years to make it different? Popular tastes have changed, certainly, but our voices haven't. The music of Bach, Handel, Haydn, Mozart, Donizetti, Bellini, and Rossini will be sung for many years to come. Therefore, there will be a constant demand for singers who can perform it.

Your throat must be free of all tension in order to sing coloratura. To enable a voice to respond automatically and freely, the same principles of letting notes be light and loose for higher pitches must be observed. A student once exclaimed, "It's like looking for something that isn't there!" The opposite, of course, is true. You will discover how sounds can be released through their natural endowment. As an action is repeated, it grows easier. Soon a response will be conditioned and you will find that your body produces tones for you. Your voice will teach you how to sing.

THE MUSCLES INVOLVED WITH COLORATURA

Many muscles are involved in adjusting the larynx for phonation. Each muscle is made up of a number of muscle fibers and each of these fibers is activated by a separate nerve fiber. A nerve has what is known as an *activation threshold*—that is, a level of excitability at which the nerve fiber will respond (Tokay, 1944). For a healthy voice one must sensitize as many of these fibers as possible.

When a muscle is used, it takes a fraction of a second for it to recover. During strenuous exercise, a muscle could be temporarily unable to respond to the next nerve impulse because it didn't have enough time to get the oxygen required to counteract the amount of lactic acid formed during use. Tension could be the culprit that prevents that new impulse from getting through.

This is one of the reasons that coloratura is so valuable in voice training. The voice moves from note to note quickly, activating new muscle fibers and releasing others. This allows for an exchange of oxygen without a buildup of fatigue. At the same time, you are exercising a range of impulses that activate many muscle fibers and therefore contribute to their growth and responsiveness. Coloratura conditions reflexive action in the muscles.

Again, quoting Martha Graham, "technique is a language that makes strain impossible!" (p. 249). Athletes prepare their muscles for performance by going through stages of stretch and light movement that are gradually increased to bring about stimulation of a maximum number of muscle fibers. The singer prepares with daily warm-ups followed by exercises of increasing difficulty as he or she progresses.

CONDITIONING AND TRAINING FOR COLORATURA

The miracle for the singer/athlete is that the vocal folds adjust automatically for a pitch just by thinking. Nothing will help you become more aware of how this happens than exercise in coloratura. Eliminate pressure from the breath and the surrounding extrinsic muscles of the larynx. Keep your mouth, jaw, and tongue free and mobile. You will soon find that good tone release leads to good resonance, which enhances the carrying power of the voice.

Good technique is what makes a great performance so exciting. Many have a glimpse along the way of what might be, but few have the discipline to carry it out. It takes great dedication and patience. Just as with other dimensions of the voice, agility takes time to develop. Master the simple scales before you move on to the more complicated. It is challenging and stimulating to move on to more and more difficult exercises. The reward that agility brings in increased vocal control is immeasurable.

If you attempt to *make* any of this happen, you will simply frustrate nature's design. The harder you try, the less it will work. In Chapter I on Primal Sound, you discovered what your voice can do when not trying for any particular quality. Once you become aware of what happens automatically, you can condition it—train it by repetition, just as athletes train their legs and body for running or jumping. Here, as with the athlete, we are working to establish kinesthetic responses. By moving quickly from one pitch to another, the muscles do not have a chance to grab, but must produce a new note and immediately release the old. Precise pitch thinking is a part of this training. Exercises should be done more slowly at first, until the scale pattern is firmly in mind. Then the speed can be gradually increased, but only to the degree that clear pitches can be articulated.

As you progress in the development of technical mastery, you will learn to let your body take over the task of execution. Breath connection is a whole-body strategy for maintaining a constant average of subglottal pressure. The physiological process is too complex for the well-trained singer to think about while performing. The mind of the artist must be free to think of what needs to be expressed musically and poetically. Technique is a means to an end, not an end in itself. Exercises XVIII through XXVIc in the appendix are designed to help you develop this skill.

Start with the exercises you can perform easily. All new scales should begin lightly. Energy will come by itself as you develop automatic responses. If the ideas expressed in the previous chapter on range and registers were not clear to you, you will have difficulty improving your agility. However, the exercises used to improve agility can lead to new possibilities in both range and the blending of registers. This is because good coloratura is based on the principle that each and every note has its own adjustment and color. Remember how the quality of tone changes in all musical instruments as notes move from one part of the range to another. Have confidence that no matter how different the pitches may sound to you, someone else hears them only as highs and lows of the same voice.

THE ART OF TRILLING

A trill was one of the most basic goals of the early masters of singing. It is a skill that has to be practiced very slowly over a long period of time before it can be executed with a distinct identity of two separate pitches. Most so-called trills that we hear today are no more than wide wobbles around the designated note. Half-note trills come first, then the whole-note trill. The secret of a successful trill is to develop the sensation that the notes are being suspended from the upper pitch like loops from a rod. To that end, exercises are given that regularly stress the upper note and loosely release the lower, almost as if you were bouncing between the two notes. This is what is meant by the instruction to do the trill from above. (See Exercises XXVII–XXVIII in the appendix.)

It may take several years to master a proper trill. The greatest patience is needed. Practice a little each day, working steadily until you have the sensation that the notes are springing back and forth by themselves. It is reported that Jenny Lind suddenly discovered how to trill by watching a bird sing. She noticed the feathers moving at the bird's throat and realized that she must completely release everything so that it could happen by itself. We can't hear Jenny Lind's voice, but we can hear that of Nellie Melba, who accomplished not only good half and whole note trills, but also mastered a trill of a minor third, which can be distinctly heard on her recording of "Sweet Bird" from Handel's *L'Allegro*.

I demonstrate some of the above exercises on the accompanying disc. It takes much "play" to work them into your voice, but the exercises show what can be done if you keep working at it.

THE KEY TO ENHANCING YOUR AGILITY

It is futile to argue that everyone can reach the same level of achievement. If this were so, everyone would be an Olympic champion. Regardless of where you start, the goal is to gain as complete a development as possible. Strive to improve flexibility; it is hard work, but whoever said learning was easy? Like mastery of any physical challenge the end result appears to be very easy but the training that is required to make it appear that way is often very taxing. The healthy ingredient in agility is the automatic release that it brings to the art of singing. *Think* what you want to sing and remove all interference so that you can *let* it happen. You then must learn to *trust* the result.

REFERENCES

Graham, M. (1991). *Blood memory*. New York: Washington Square Press. p. 4
    & p. 249.

Tokay, E. (1944). *Fundamentals of physiology*. New York: Barnes & Noble.

VIII

■

RESONANCE AND POWER

// **I** want more power," explained a lawyer who had come to Timothy Gallwey (1976) for a lesson on his tennis serve. Gallwey, who follows the Zen philosophy of letting your body teach your mind, proceeded to take his student through a series of exercises designed to release his body's energy, with never a word about force. I highly recommend his books as supplemental reading for voice students.

WHAT IS POWER?

Power! Power! What is meant by all this emphasis on power? Does it mean that singers must try to make their voices BIG? Let's make this clear right away: You do not need a "big" voice to "fill the house." If you do not possess a big voice, perhaps you are blessed; people with big voices often have great difficulty learning to sing softly. The size of your voice is given to you at birth. The task of every singer is to learn how to develop the *carrying quality* of the voice. A student with a naturally big voice frequently has a temperament that goes with it and wants to do things in a big way. It is good to remember at this stage that singing as we perform it today is a human invention. It takes great patience and much time to develop the potential of the larynx for the many tasks imposed upon it.

In physics, *intensity* refers to how far molecules move and with what energy. Perceptually, this is experienced as *loudness*.

In music, the term intensity has a variety of meanings. For example, a musician may use the term when speaking of emotional effect as well as loudness.

Carrying quality can be deceptive. Unfortunately, you cannot hear your own voice the way other people hear it. Even trained musicians are sometimes fooled by the acoustics of a small room. Gatti-Casazza, director of the Metropolitan Opera from 1908 to 1935, gave Kirsten Flagstad only a one year contract because he was not sure her voice was big enough to fill the house. He had auditioned her in a relatively small room in Switzerland and was not prepared for the effect of the rich overtones in her voice when she sang in the auditorium of the old Met—and Flagstad's voice was not always considered big. She sang many lyric roles in her younger days. It was only when she was nearly 40 that the fullness of her voice materialized. It has been noted many times that the great Wagnerian and Verdian voices did not come into their prime until the artists were in their late thirties. This is true of men as well as women.

Our ears are constructed to protect us from the intensity of our own sound (see Chapter XVIII), which is why others do not hear us as we hear ourselves. You must learn to trust that the sounds you produce have ample intensity. Listen to what your teacher and others tell you. Also, tape-record your voice to prove the point to yourself. It is very common, especially among sopranos, to question whether the high tones can be heard, since they can barely hear the tones themselves. A soprano feels that she is hardly doing anything at all.

Another reason for not listening to yourself is that what you hear will vary depending on where you sing. Even within an auditorium, different locations on stage or different costumes—especially hats—will make a difference in what you hear. The relation of your position to the orchestra will also affect what you hear and may make you want to compete with the orchestra. You must be guided by proprioception, the "sixth sense of singing." Your inner hearing, sensing, and feeling are the prime monitors of what you are producing.

A young tenor who came to me had a tendency to oversing his high notes. He had never been taught to exercise his Register 3 voice. Having a rather large, athletic physique and the mistaken attitude about falsetto that so many young men have, he was reluctant to practice those notes, but did so just to humor me. About a year later he was engaged as tenor soloist in Beethoven's Ninth Symphony for a series of four concerts. When the rehearsals started, he was just getting over a cold, so he decided to use only his upper voice for the high passages. He felt this was no time to compete for volume with the other soloists. A friend taped the rehearsal from the back of the auditorium. To his amazement, his voice carried better than any of the others. He determined he would only sing that way from then on, and has since performed Heldentenor roles in Europe. Although he was thinking "upper voice," he was actually blending it with his lower voice, which produces full high tones.

The distinguished Danish bass, Aage Haugland, performs the role of Baron Ochs in *Der Rosenkavalier* with enviable dynamic control ranging from loud bluster to delicate pianissimos. This is in a range from C below the staff to a high G#. Haugland started as a counter tenor and today places great value on exercising the falsetto range of his voice. This certainly says something about integrating all parts of the voice, not only for range, but also for volume.

UNDERSTANDING RESONANCE

Size, resonance and carrying power are interconnected. Webster (Merriam-Webster, 1981) defines *resonance* as the relationship between two bodies, or "reinforcement and prolongation of a sound by reflection or by vibration of other bodies." Increase the mass of the resonator and the amount of resonance will increase. Depending on the size, shape, and substance of the resonator, it can make the various energies of sound amplify differently. When sound is rebounded, there are reinforcements and cancellations of the various frequencies.

The chief resonators are the pharynx (the throat above the larynx) and the mouth. Moveable or adjustable parts of these resonators include the pharynx itself, the tongue, the jaw, the soft palate, and the lips. The pyriform sinuses, trachea, chest, and the whole body also act to some degree as resonators. Vibrations can be measured from the toes, and you feel them from the top of the head by simply placing your hand there. Physical differences in these resonators have much to do with the qualities that distinguish one voice from another.

The work you have been doing in letting an airflow activate the vocal folds is now paying off in another way. Sundberg (1981) reports that "flow phonation generates the loudest vowel sound." Like so many other features of singing, you must be free of any unnecessary tension so that resonance, too, can happen. If you have been able to assimilate the materials up to this point, you are ready to move forward to one of the final technical facets of voice production. A naturally full voice can have a muffled quality, or a relatively small voice a penetrating quality, depending on the mixture of the resonance areas involved in the tone.

Closing off some of our resonance chambers by a bunched tongue, for example, can result in a pinched sound as well as the cancellation of some of the overtones. If there is to be resonance, there must be freedom and room for it to work. A relaxed laryngeal position is not only beneficial in ways already mentioned but also provides a longer resonating column in the pharynx. As it lowers, it enhances the conical shape in the throat, radiating upward and outward from the glottis.

As you tend to widen your throat in commencing a yawn, the larynx lowers and the pyriform sinuses, which lie on either side of the larynx, expand. The resonance of these sinuses has been measured by Winckel (1971) at between 2800 and 3000 Hz, the characteristic "ring" of the voice! It is this quality that permits a voice to be heard over an orchestra, since no orchestral instrument has strong resonances in this range. A modern symphony orchestra has a peak of around 450 Hz.

By removing the high overtones from a recording of a voice singing with an orchestra, the voice is not heard. When the overtones are restored, the voice "rides over the orchestra." Of course, if the orchestra plays too loudly, especially the brasses, it is more difficult for the voice.

We find in the chapter on physics that a tone has what is known as a fundamental and overtones. These are expressed in frequencies or vibrations per second. A *formant* is a group of frequencies that changes in value according to the vowel being sung and the enhancement of certain overtones. By changing the adjustable parts of the resonators, we intensify some overtones and dampen others. We identify these changing qualities as different vowels plus the amplification of energy in a frequency region which occurs at between 2800 and 3200 Hz (Bunch, 1982; Sundberg, 1977; Vennard, 1967). That ring is known as the *singer's formant.*

When the base of the tongue is relaxed, the larynx can rest low and help to create a freer space at the back of the throat. If the soft palate rises, this assists in creating pharyngeal space and, by reflex action, helps the larynx to rest low. All this results in a feeling that the tone is not only darker, but further back. Vocalizing on "oh" (o) or "oo" (u) helps lower the larynx because of the sucking reflex of the lip formation. A sensation of ring or nasal resonance begins to develop at the same time. The resonance sensations are by-products of the correct function in other areas and are not prime objectives in themselves. When resonance is properly developed, you have the sensation that all the vowel sounds emanate from some area in the middle of your head, perhaps just behind the soft palate.

These sensations can be a guide for producing voice but should not be sought out for themselves in early study. I am definitely not of the school that seeks to "*place* the voice in the mask" or any other place. Such an endeavor would be putting the cart before the horse.

Sound travels at the rate of 1,088 feet per second at sea level—and 0°C temperature—more than three times the length of a football field. Can you imagine trying to "direct" or "place" a sound which travels at that rate from within the confines of the pharynx and the mouth?

Sound also travels in spherical waves, like light from a lightbulb. As pressure of interfering tension is released, the tone is bigger through the increased resonance made possible by the free interplay of the space areas in the throat, mouth, and head. To help experience and release the forces of resonance, let everything in your body be free, down to the very soles of your feet. If you then take an easy, low breath with a sense that you start the tone almost before you finish taking your breath, you can begin to feel what is meant by the expression "floating the tone." It rides out on a gentle flow of air and it has resonance.

FINDING YOUR RESONANCE POTENTIAL

The variables of muscular interplay and breath flow rate should be developed carefully. Caution must always be taken not to overload the larynx by the greater power of the lungs. Remember that as muscles are exercised, they grow. It is that simple. You must learn to let your voice lead you to discover its new strength and not reach out to try to "make" it before the proper conditions have been established.

What a teacher hears as potential and what it takes to develop it are two different things. The following story is a good illustration. A student came to me when she was 15 without having studied previously. As she progressed, I realized I was working with a young, full-voiced mezzo-soprano with a range of three octaves: C one octave below the staff to high C. She was physically strong and healthy. It all fitted together.

When she was 19 she entered a regional National Association of Teachers of Singing (NATS) competition for students aged 19 to 25. After long deliberation, the judges awarded her second place. First place was awarded to a 25-year-old tenor named Jon Humphrey, a most worthy winner. Every teacher present who spoke to the young lady commented on what a fine dramatic soprano she was going to become!

This student went away to college and, incidentally, studied with a teacher who worked to develop her as a dramatic soprano. At the end of the year, the young lady returned to me, but it took a whole year of corrective exercises to free her from the excessive pressure and tension she had acquired in that one year of study and to return to her lush, easy three-octave range she had before she went away.

This student had perfect pitch. Because of this, she told me after a period of study that she was never sure "which way to go" when she sang B or B-flat in the middle of the staff. This placed her in the category of mezzo or contralto, which could be recognized when she sang low. Yet, her top range was so free that it sounded like a soprano. Many accomplished mezzos demonstrate these same qualities. Keep tessitura in mind when dealing with a potentially big voice.

NASAL RESONANCE

The quality you feel as nasal resonance is very desirable. It is associated with the ring in the voice and is created when (a) full use is made of the resonators, (b) your throat is free from tensions, and (c) you have a good glottal adjustment. Although nasal resonance is a sensation in the area of the turbinates, scientific investigations have proven that strong resonance is not produced there. Nasal resonance and nasality are two different things. Nasality results when the soft palate lowers when vowel sounds are sung, and is not a desirable quality other than in certain French vowels.

As you begin to sense a ring in your voice, give attention to "riding" it, much as violinists learn to ride the overtones of their instrument by the way they manage their bowing. Violinists have also discovered that their instruments produce bigger tones when undue pressure is removed. Remember that perfecting technique means finding a manner of execution which produces the best results with the least effort.

GOOD RESONANCE COMES WITH TIME AND TRAINING

With proper exercise over a period of time, your vocal folds develop a better tonus or firmness. No young, untrained singer has the strength in his or her vocal folds that a mature singer has. Many years ago Bell Laboratories took pictures of the vocal folds of an untrained singer and a trained singer, each producing the same pitch. The pictures were made with their new camera, which could shoot 5,000 frames per second. When this was played back at the normal rate, the motion was greatly slowed so that details invisible to the naked eye could be studied. What especially impressed me was that the folds of the untrained singer would separate quite widely in each cycle of vibration, whereas the folds of the trained singer hardly parted at all. The trained singer's voice, therefore, produced a firm, ringing sound with little air escape. The untrained singer's voice was quite breathy, with little or no ring.

As the muscles of the larynx grow stronger, they make a better closure and therefore create a greater resistance to the expiratory flow of air. Let me hasten to point out, however, that a trained singer makes no effort to hold, push, or squeeze his vocal folds together! The folds are extremely sensitive to emotion and/or a thought of sound and respond by coming into position for phonation automatically. Training sensitizes the folds to make the proper adjustments for the desired sounds in both speech and singing. The right kind of exercise over a period of time brings about a firmness and strength in the muscles themselves. You discover that your voice seems stronger and that the folds are making better connection to the breath.

At this stage of development, a proper understanding of breath connection frees the larynx from undue stress. Review the experiments of Leanderson and Sundberg, in Chapter III, on posture and breathing. Remember that as the vocal folds adjust for higher pitches there is automatically a greater pressure due to the greater tension in the laryngeal adjustments. This utilizes a greater amount of energy stored in your lungs when you take a breath. (See Venturi Effect in Chapter XV.) Increases in the activity of those intrinsic muscles of the larynx which increase tension in the vocal folds occur with increases in vocal intensity (Colton, 1988). Thus loud and/or high notes will fatigue the voice more quickly.

The automatic breath pressure that takes place when you suddenly call "Hey!" has already been described. In soft singing there is a noticeable activation of the diaphragm that prevents the expiratory flow of air from being too great. The "messa di voce" (Exercise XXX, in the appendix) will heighten your awareness of this kind of breath connection. I have worked with singers who could sing high C from pianissimo to double forte and back again with perfect coordination. (Exercises XXIX–XXXIV; listen to the compact disc illustration.)

The variables of muscular interplay and breath connection should be developed carefully over a long period of time. Never overload the larynx with the greater power of the lungs. Let your voice lead you to discover its new strength. Don't reach out and try to make it. Proper conditioning will bring out the ring and carrying power for you.

Investigations by the Chinese teacher and scientific researcher Professor Shiqian Wang (1983) show that this ring in the voice can also be produced if tones are sung with the larynx high, as is done by Chinese male opera singers. This is in contrast to the low larynx position recommended by Western teachers. There seems to be no harm to the vocal folds. The quality produced is the prime difference and could be considered a cultural choice. Western audiences seem to prefer the darker color which results from tones produced with a low larynx, over the bright quality that results from tones produced with a high larynx. The low larynx is a must for the integration of the different registers of the voice desired in the European tradition. The high larynx position produces the quality used by many popular singers.

WORKING WITH THE ORCHESTRA

In most lyric music, the orchestration is light and, with a good conductor, there is no problem. A good conductor is needed in all instances. Far too often the conductor does not understand the human voice and its potential as an instrument. This applies to many church choir directors, as well as to high school and college choral conductors, composers, and stage directors. Many orchestral conductors have not spent as much time getting to know the voice as they have getting to know the orchestral instruments. The human voice did not come out of a factory.

The different locations of orchestra pits in opera houses make a difference in how the singer on stage perceives his or her own voice. From Wagner's Festspielhaus in Bayreuth, where the orchestra is under the stage, to the Metropolitan Opera at Lincoln Center in New York City, where the orchestra is entirely exposed and out in front of the stage, there are all sorts of variations. The problems involved are really the responsibility of the conductor. The singers' responsibility is to thoroughly know their own voice and not change the way they use it based on orchestra location and concert hall acoustics. I have witnessed some disastrous results from artists who tried to overcome poor acoustics by singing louder. In the words of Maria Callas, "There is the danger of trying too hard and ruining something beautiful by losing control or exaggerating" (Ardoin, 1987, p. 10).

If power were the important criterion many feel it to be, we would never have known the artistry, technical skill, and beauty in the voices of Titto Schippa, Jussi Bjoerling, or Joseph Schmidt. Read about them. Listen to their records. The artist Elizabeth Schumann had a light, small voice, but it carried. This was also true of Bidu Sayou and Judith Blegen. The tragedy is that so many voices are ruined on the altar of POWER! If a voice has size and power, one does not have to make it. If a voice is naturally not big, it can develop concentration of tone and carrying quality, but it can never be a dramatic voice, as most people think of power. Think in terms of concentrated tone, not power.

TRAINING FOR POWER

In 1954, it was my privilege to serve as an analyst at a convetion of the National Association of Teachers of singing. The convention attendees were divided into several groups, each assigned a different topic for exploration. Our group probed the subject "How to Train for Power." It was my job to keep our group on the track and then try to glean guidelines from the findings of the majority. Two former presidents of NATS were members of this group, as well as other distinguished teachers. We arrived at a unanimous set of findings which have never been published. I believe them to be of great interest and include them here.

FINDINGS OF THE COMMITTEE ON
HOW TO TRAIN FOR POWER

**National Convention of the
National Association of Teachers of Singing
Chattanooga, Tennessee
December 27–30, 1954**

1. We understand *power* to mean the development of full, rich, free, resonant tone to the greatest potential of the individual voice.

We recognize that there is a great variance in the degree of power in different voices, but it is our concept that the term *power* may be applied to a lyric voice as well as to a dramatic voice.

We believe one should not train for power as a separate entity; however, optimum power is desirable in a well-trained voice.

2. We hold that the statement of laws and precepts upon which vocal pedagogy may be based, as set forth by the National Association of Teachers of Singing, is indispensable to any pattern of training which has power as its objective. These include the following precepts:

    a. Posture
    b. Breathing
    c. Release
    d. Resonance
    e. Vowel and consonant formation
    f. Diction
    g. Pronunciation and articulation

3. We hold that no single dynamic of the voice should be isolated in its development from the full range of dynamics.

4. In regard to vowel formation, the intensity of vowel formation must be maintained as the power is increased.

In loud or "forced" singing, facial contortions and straining neck muscles are often observed. Maintaining an intense but free vowel formation is regarded as a safeguard. A proper release of interfering muscles of the throat must accompany an increase of breath pressure to maintain a powerful tone. Power must never be achieved at the expense of tonal beauty.

5. One must guard against imitation of dramatic singing.

Attempting to endow one's voice with a certain quality, range, or volume by artificial means merely results in vocal strain and its consequences.

6. In powerful singing the artist is always the master of his elements not the servant.

Dramatic tones sung in a display of sheer vocal power and showmanship destroy the artistic interpretation of the song.

7. The voice teacher must know the physiological capacity of the vocal instrument in order to safeguard it throughout its entire period of training.

One of the most valuable elements, often overlooked, is that the voice needs rest as well as exercise.

8. We feel that power is the result of training over an extended period of time.

We must recognize that the vocal cords are muscles and require care and time in order to reach their maximum development. You can plant a rose today but you cannot pick a blossom tomorrow.

Moderator: **Paul Peterson**
Analyst: **Oren Brown**
Recorder: **Ruth Scott Parker**

I believe that the Committee's findings, for the most part, hold true today. With our increased understanding of vowel modification, guidelines for achieving point 4 might be worded a bit differently. Perhaps it would read, "In regard to vowel formation, it is desirable to maintain as much of the vowel's identity as possible as the power is increased."

As an analogy of how an end-product of dependable strength can result from a small beginning, I like to think of how the cables of the George Washington Bridge were constructed. One wire, suspended between two towers, was sufficiently strong to support a small machine which could carry a second wire, slowly winding it around the first as it traveled from tower to tower. This process was continued until the huge and powerful cables that exist today were completed. At no time did the engineers test the incomplete work with an overload. Such folly would have forced them to start all over again.

Another analogy is that of the fairytale princess locked in a tower with no means of escape except a spool of thread. By holding on to one end, she could drop the other end to her prince waiting below. He could then attach a stronger thread which the princess could then pull up to her balcony. By gradually increasing the strength of the thread he attached, she could eventually gain a rope of sufficient length and strength to hold her.

I love these stories because they so closely parallel developing a voice from the top down in a manner that allows those upper fibrous adjustments to counterbalance the bulk and strength of the lower muscular adjustments in full and complete phonation. How often, though, strength is put to the test too soon, and strain introduced, forcing the student to go back and start from the beginning. Far fetched, you say? Think about it.

I hope you have deduced from this discussion on resonance that it has a great deal to do with what is called power. Vitality of tone, concentration, or focus are the objectives in all study, but they must be achieved without undue stress or excessive manipulation. There are those who believe that vocalizing on the "ee" [i] vowel can help in producing a concentrated tone in some cases. Good laryngeal tonus and coordination are the objective. A firm tonus is not possible in young, untrained voices, and should not be expected until a voice has reached an advanced stage of technical development.

Understanding the source of your sound and why it works the way it does can put to rest all thoughts of trying to *make* a sound. When you push any mechanism, including the voice, to its physiological limits, control of the output will be less precise than it would be with a more conservative approach. A shout and a singing tone have very different qualities. A cry of alarm or fright might have a very high frequency, but would not be consistent in quality with sung tones of the same frequency. Such a cry would be, therefore, an undesirable means of producing high frequency.

Yes, we want to have resonance and power as part of the technique of singing. With the exercises and safeguards presented in this chapter, growth will come about naturally, rather than being superimposed on the voice. There is no set time schedule. Some discover this relatively early in their study, whereas others do not discover what can happen for many years. I know of no shortcuts.

It is by *thinking* correctly that you can *let* growth take place in a natural way. There is no area in vocal production where you have to *trust* the results more than in learning to develop resonance and power.

REFERENCES

Ardoin, J. (1987). *Callas at Juilliard*, New York: Knopf.
Bunch, M. (1982). *Dynamics of the singing voice*, New York: Springer-Verlag.

Colton, R. (1988). *Physiological mechanisms of vocal frequency control; the role of tension,* in Journal of Voice, Vol. 2, #3, New York: Raven Press, (pp. 208–220).

Gallwey, W.T. (1976). *Inner tennis,* New York: Random House, (p. 17).

Merriam-Webster's *Eghth Collegiate Dictionary.* (1981). Springfield, Ma: Merriam-Webster.

Sundberg, J. (1977, March). *The acoustics of the singing voice,* Scientific American, (p. 82)

Sundberg, J. (1981). *The voice as a sound generator, research aspects of singing,* in Royal Swedish Academy of Music, 33.

Vennard, W. (1967). *Singing: The mechanism and technic,* New York: Carl Fischer.

Wang, S. (1983). *Bright timbre, acoustic features and larynx position,* Paper presented at 105th meeting of the Acoustical Society of America.

Winckel, F. (1971). *How to measure the effectiveness of stage singers' voices,* Pholia Phonistica, 23.

IX

■

GROWTH AND MATURATION

About 95% of promising young voices that start out on a career fail because the laryngeal phonatory mechanism will not stand the long, grueling ordeal of vocal training.

Though faulty method may be ruinous, voices can be forever ruined by excessive singing by any method.

Prevention is better than cure. Laryngeal muscles must have rest.

These three quotations are from the famous throat specialist Chevalier Jackson (1940, p. 434). He was writing about a very severe condition called *myasthenia laryngis*, a disability of the phonatory laryngeal muscles from overuse (Dorland, 1951).

A young businessman was referred to me for treatment of vocal nodules. As I explained how overuse of his voice could put strain on his vocal muscles, he said, "I know exactly what you mean." "How do you know?" I inquired. This was his story. When he was in high school he showed unusual promise as a baseball pitcher. His father was an athletic coach. The boy would work out at home by throwing a baseball at a bucket as target, the bucket having been set at the distance of home plate from the pitcher's mound. Everyone thought he would become the next Dizzy Dean, a famous pitcher. When he entered college with a generous athletic scholarship, he was placed on a vigorous training program through the fall and winter in preparation for the spring season. But when spring arrived, his arm was "burnt out," an expression for over-use of an athlete's muscle. His promising career was over, finished, irretrievably gone. His understanding of what it meant to use a muscle too long or too heavily gave him an excellent chance of improving his voice, which, fortunately, had not been used to the same excess as his pitching arm.

BASIC PRINCIPLES OF GROWTH AND MATURATION

Vocal growth and maturation have so many variables that it is only possible to state some of the basic principles. At the heart of the subject is the fact that the vocal folds were not placed in your body primarily for making sound. (See Chapter XVI, Laryngeal Anatomy and Physiology.) Although there can be a child prodigy in piano or violin, you can't expect the same for voice because the larynx grows and changes the voice over time. More than that, you must keep in mind that the laryngeal muscles are very small and need to be exercised a little at a time over a comparatively long period. Under the best conditions, it could take between five and ten years to develop a vocal athlete.

I remember a voice therapy patient who, as I gave her exercises to do a little at a time, kept saying to me, "I ought to have known that. That is what Auntie used to do." It turned out that her aunt was a dramatic soprano named Eleanora de Cisneros (1878–1934) who had sung at the Metropolitan Opera, La Scala, and many other places. This great opera singer, with a reputation for a very large voice, had a routine of practicing in very short periods, but a number of times a day. She also practiced quite lightly most of the time.

COMPARISON OF YOUTHS' AND ADULTS' VOICES

In his biography of Nellie Melba, Wechsberg (1961) quotes Melba: "I implore young singers not to attempt to sing roles which are beyond their power" (p. 255). Wechsberg, himself, said, "The world's great opera houses are populated with singers who ruined their voices prematurely by singing parts that are beyond their power" (p. 255).

Bear in mind that the average human body has not finished growing until age 21. There may be variance on either side, a few displaying maturity as young as 16 and others not until they are 24 or 25, but you can't expect an adult sound from bodies that are not fully matured.

I knew a young tenor who was given the role of Sigmund in Wagner's *Die Walkure* to study at age 17, and a baritone who was handed the Prologue from *Pagliacci* at his first lesson! Teachers who assign this kind of material to immature voices should not be teaching singing.

You don't study arias to learn how to sing. You learn how to sing so that you may study arias. But let's examine what is the same for both young and adult voices.

1. Each has a larynx which can produce tones over a range of two to three octaves.
2. Each produces a pitch by thinking it and allowing the vocal folds to adjust automatically.
3. Each needs to learn to bring breathing under the willed control within a framework of good posture.
4. Each needs to learn to use that upper part of the range which is not used in ordinary conversation.
5. Each needs to discover what the voice can do without any excess pushing or straining for loud tones or for range.
6. Each must learn that his voice has its own unique quality and that, therefore, he should not try to imitate the voice of any other individual, whether heard on records, radio, television, film, or in person.
7. Each must learn to trust how his own voice feels when he sings and not depend on hearing himself. (Is it easy? Can he sing without his throat getting tired? etc.)
8. Each must learn that just because someone else can do something doesn't mean that he can do the same thing. There is the fact of individual capacity.
9. Each must learn that to be good at anything takes time and regular practice.
10. Each must learn that he can't do anything with his voice that he can't conceive in his mind.
11. Each uses the same vocal folds for singing that are used for speech; therefore, bad use in speech will adversely affect singing, and vice-versa.
12. Each must accept the fact that it is better to do too little than too much.

We should also consider what differentiates young from adult voices:

1. Young singers have greater lung pressure in proportion to the size of their larynx than do adults.

2. Unchanged children's voices are essentially the same for both boys and girls, whereas in adults the male voice is roughly an octave lower in range than the female voice.
3. The quality of children's voices is light, lyric, and sometimes by nature a bit breathy, whereas the adult voice takes on a much fuller and darker quality.
4. The adult's voice is capable of developing much greater intensity than the child's voice
5. The adult's voice can express a much wider range of emotion than the child's voice.

Because young and adult voices have so much in common, the elements of maturation must constantly be kept in mind. A great deal will depend on the individual and the type of voice. A lyric can often start much younger than a heavier voice. Roberta Peters was 19 when she made her Metropolitan Opera debut. Men start when they are older because their voices change so dramatically at puberty. The age at which an individual begins study also makes a difference in when he or she starts to sing professionally. There have been great singers who did not commence study until they were in their mid twenties.

A big, dramatic voice usually begins to show potential much sooner than it is ready to perform the dramatic repertoire. But, if a student has no bad habits, exceptional ability may be displayed quite early. I remember hearing the baritone Donald Gramm sing very beautifully at age 17. I also heard Grace Bumbry sing "O don fatale" at age 15! She continued to study for some eight years before she started to sing professionally, however.

People sometimes think that because an exceptional child like Adelina Patti (1843–1919) made her first public appearance at age 7, all children should be able to do the same thing. This is like saying that every child should be able to compose like Mozart or dance like Shirley Temple.

Ernestine Schumann-Heink (1861–1936), Conchita Supervia (1895–1936), and Patti (all mentioned in Chapter VII) continued to sing way beyond childhood. Supervia's career was cut short by her premature death, but we have recordings of Patti that were made when she was in her sixties. Schumann-Heink appeared in a movie at age 75.

LAWS OF MUSCLE DEVELOPMENT APPLY TO VOICE

In 1988, Donald Henahan wrote a feature article for the Sunday *New York Times* entitled "Why Singers Don't Set Records." He pointed out that mechanical assistance such as "microphones and amplifiers have contributed to the deterioration of vocal technique, the 'sine qua non' of vocal art." He claimed that this was because audiences that have been exposed since childhood to greatly amplified but relatively untrained voices now accept almost any sound from the throat.

I have often compared the relationship of a voice teacher and his student to that of a race horse trainer and his horse. The horse has no idea of how fast it can go, how far or how soon. If the trainer "gives the horse his head," weeks or months of training will be lost because what has been developed will be undone. The wise trainer gets to know each horse and allows it to add new tasks only when it has been conditioned to begin them. If only voice teachers studied each student with the care and consideration a good horse trainer gives to his horse!

There is the saying that you should not judge a book by its cover. Certainly, you should not try to estimate a voice by physique. A young man, built like a football player, came to see me for study after completing his master's degree at a large university. He had performed as a baritone soloist a number of times during his college years. Shortly after he commenced his study with me, he developed a severe cold. I referred him to an otolaryngologist who phoned me during the examination to report that this young man of 24 had a larynx the size of a child's. We could not expect his voice to become big—which is what the young man had come to me for and what I had hoped could happen for him. You can't change Mother Nature so you had better know the facts and go along with her. This student chose to channel his musical talents and vocal knowledge into becoming a choral conductor.

Your voice must follow the same laws of muscle development that apply to other muscles of the body. This is because the muscles that control the laryngeal adjustments are very small. Just as other muscles grow by the application of proper exercise, so the voice will grow over a period of time. Each voice has its own capacity for growth, however. The number of muscle fibers will vary from individual to individual—even from one side of the larynx to the other.

I had a 22-year-old student who experienced great difficulty learning to blend his Register 3 voice with his Register 2. An examination by a throat specialist revealed a marked asymmetry of the larynx. It would shift to the left whenever he started to sing. It seems that he had studied the flute from age 7 to 18, at which time he decided to study singing. The muscles in the left side of his neck were disproportionately strong from turning his head in that direction for so many years of flute playing. To correct this, I had him do all his singing with his head turned in the other direction for two years. Finally, his voice behaved in a normal manner and he could blend his registers. This can also happen if a student has studied violin at an early age.

Some have argued that a "natural" voice needs nothing more than appropriate music. On the contrary, I observe that a natural voice needs training based on the physical laws of vocal production to blossom into a healthy singing instrument. There has never been any great performing art without great technique.

In an interview with Will Crutchfield (1991), Marilyn Horne had this to say about voice training: "Most of the young singers I hear simply have not been taught properly. They have no idea of breath control and all they can do is push. I would say that this goes for 90% of Americans, and now I hear it all over Europe, too."

There has been much investigation of vibrato, the vibrating quality of a tone. I have found that excessive vibrato, commonly referred to as a "wobble," is often caused by applying too much pressure for dramatic effect or a big tone. If too much weight or "dark" color is carried up from the bottom, your voice will eventually develop a wobble. Excessive laryngeal tension can be transmitted to the immediate surrounding muscles, and a shaking jaw or pulsating tongue can be seen. You should not use more of the lower (Register 2) heavy mechanism than can be balanced by the lighter, upper adjustments (Register 3), as explained in Chapter V on Range and Registers. As you get older, if you do not regularly exercise the Number 3 Register, there is the danger that a wobble will develop. I have observed this often in men's and women's voices.

In contrast to an excessive vibrato, a good vibrato will contain intensity as well as pitch variation. The intensity alterations are the result of the periodic amplification and rarification of the overtones with the fundamental. I believe that the pitch vibrato results from the action of the nerve impulses as they act on the intrinsic muscles of the larynx in adjustments for frequency.

Spanish singers may tend toward a fast vibrato; the English oratorio school favors a straight tone. Variances of vocal timbre from race to race and from nationality to nationality may be influenced by both language and culture. Cultural differences explain variations in vibrato to some degree.

DEVELOPMENT OF VOICE IN THE LATER YEARS

In 1986, Jane E. Brody wrote a pair of articles for *The New York Times* on aging. In these she wrote, "Researchers are finding that moderate exercise can not only retard the effects of aging but can actually reverse them" (p. C14). She went on to say that "proper exercise, even into the 80s and beyond, has been shown to significantly deter the deterioration of bodily functions that traditionally accompany aging" (p. C1). Safe levels of exercise are cautioned, with the recommendation that you see your doctor and that you start in slowly, keeping your limits in mind.

In the spring of 1992, Marta Eggerth was the star of the evening in a gala performance at Carnegie Hall in honor of the 100th birthday of Richard Tauber (1892–1948). With tones as clear as a bell, she brought down the house at the age of 79.

Hugues Cuenod, the Swiss tenor, made his debut at the Met at age 87! Roland Hayes was still giving recitals in his eighties. These examples demonstrate that when you use your voice correctly, provided that you have good health, you can sing for years. Many great artists have had careers that lasted thirty or more years.

You know the saying: "Use it or lose it." Singers with long careers keep their voices in condition by vocalizing regularly. This is especially important with respect to the upper half of the voice, which is not used in ordinary conversation. A daily routine of light exercises is a must. Brody's article on aging states in closing, "It takes many weeks to reach a peak level of conditioning, but it can be lost in a week or two of inactivity" (p. C14). I can bear witness to this by my experience of taking a "summer off," only to find that it took me from September to January to get my voice back into sufficient condition to illustrate simple exercises for my students. This happened when I was about 70 years old. Since then, I've never let more than a day or two go by without some vocalizing.

HEALTHY EXPECTATIONS OF VOCAL MATURATION

The biggest threat to the healthy growth and maturation of your voice is trying to do too much too soon. You must discover what nature intended for you, not try to make your voice into something that it isn't.

Refinements develop with experience and continue to grow over the years—even after you are performing professionally. If you have arrived at this point safely, I would tend to trust the direction of your development in the future. By "listening" to what your body tells you, you will know what feels just right and what seems to be wrong.

"Know what you know and know that you don't know what you don't know. This is the mark of one who knows" (Confucius, 551–479 BC).

Think. Keep your mind and thoughts clear about what you can expect of your voice. If you do that and learn to *let* your voice grow at its own pace, you can *trust* the result.

REFERENCES

Brody, J.E. (1986, June 10). *Aging: Studies point toward ways to slow it.* New York Times, (p. C1).

Brody, J.E. (1986, June 11). *Safe levels of exercise to help the elderly stay vigorous.* New York Times (p. C14).

Crutchfield, W. (1991, May 24). *Homespun virtues still drive a reigning diva.* New York Times, Arts & Leisure Section, (pp. 1 & 23).

Dorland, W.A. (1951). *The American illustrated medical dictionary,* (22nd ed.). Philadelphia: Saunders.

Henahan, D. (1988, March 6). *Why singers don't set records,* New York Times.

Jackson, C. (1940, September). *Myasthenia laryngis.* Archives of Otolaryngology, 32, p. 434.

Wechsberg, J. (1961). *Red plush and black velvet,* Boston: Little, Brown, (p. 255).

X

■

ARTICULATION

"__O__ __ __E__ __ A__E__I__A." These are the vowels in the first three words of one of America's best known songs. You could sing the melody with them. But what do they mean? Let's put in the consonants and leave out the vowels. "G__D BL__SS __M__R__C__." You definitely couldn't sing a melody on that. Put it all together and you could not only sing it, but know what it meant as well.

So far, you have been exercising your voice on vowels because they are the elements in language sustained by laryngeal sound. Vocal literature is made up of words, however, which are combinations of vowels and consonants. Callas compared legato singing to a telephone wire with birds perched on it. The birds represent the consonants and the wire a steady flow of tone.

The human voice is the only instrument that can communicate words. Music is said to heighten the meaning of text. But what is the purpose of text if you can't understand it? Although a mother can understand the babbling of her baby, the level of communication is very elementary. Who wants to attend a song recital and hear baby talk? Yet, what you hear is very often little better.

The communication of words imposes an added task on the vocalist: muscle mobility for articulation. Good pronunciation can make the difference between a poor performance and an excellent one. When well implemented, pronunciation adds color, energy, and interest and enhances the legato line.

In Italy one summer, a student who was struggling to learn the language turned to me and said, "Even the children can speak

Italian!" "Yes, and so can the parrots," I answered, having just passed a house where the pet bird was rattling along with great fluency.

As a child, you learned to speak by imitation. No one taught you how to breathe or how to shape the words. What you need to learn now is how to speak professionally.

Language is shape. Words are made of a series of different shapes. You are already aware of how a flow of air can give you sound. That same flow of air also provides the energy for creating consonants. The jaw, tongue, lips, soft palate, and pharynx mold the vowels and the consonants. As the space in your mouth and pharynx are formed into different shapes, the various overtones of your primal sound are enhanced or suppressed, producing qualities which are called vowels. The voice scientist recognizes the resulting composite of concentrations of energy at particular frequencies as the *vowel formant* (Ladefoged, 1962; see Figure X–1). The manner in which the articulators interrupt or resist the airflow creates a series of noises labeled *consonants*. Most consonants do not have the sustaining properties of vowels (e.g., *t* or *p*) and are called *unvoiced consonants*. Others incorporate a simultaneous sound from your larynx, (e.g., *m* or *v*) and may be sustained. This group is classified as *voiced consonants*.

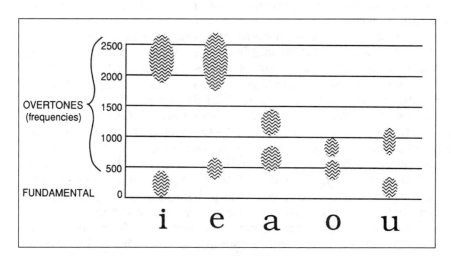

Figure X–1. Formants—approximate figures. The shape of the vocal tract determines the frequencies of the formant. The first two overtones are the most important in determining the vowel. The "color" of the vowel will change according to the exact positions of the overtones, which can vary up or down, as indicated by the boundaries around each overtone.

For purposes of analysis and study, language is broken down into single units called *phonemes*. These are represented by symbols which form what is known as the International Phonetic Alphabet (IPA). For example, [i] stands for the vowel sound we recognize as *e*. The same symbol is used for that sound in whatever language it occurs. If you know the IPA, you can learn to pronounce any language as long as it is written with IPA symbols.

If you phonate on different pitches at the same time that you shape words, you are carrying out two distinct operations simultaneously. This is the ideal (Brown, 1953). You already know that you can shape a sound without words. As an experiment, ask a friend to watch your lips as you silently count from one to five and then see if he can tell you what you said.

I like to compare the generation of speech to the image of a spotlight which would represent the source of sound, the glottis, and the origin of your primal schwa [ə]. Different colored gelatins placed alternately in front of the spotlight would then symbolize the vowels. If the colored light thus produced was subsequently given form by being passed through a variety of shaped openings, these would equate with the consonants. The final shaped, colored light would represent the word. The only missing element in this picture would be the unvoiced consonants.

Figure X–2 presents a number of IPA symbols. I have attempted to keep it as simple as possible, only representing those sounds that are used in American stage or professional English. If you master this, you should be understood by any American audience.

VOWELS

Vowels are sometimes represented by the "vowel triangle" (Figure X–3). In this image, the vowels are placed in a sequence which has been called "closed" at each end and progresses toward the "open" middle. Beginning with [i] (as in *eve*), they are shaped principally by your tongue and from the other end [u] (as in *ooze*) by your lips. The one vowel that does not fit into this series is [ɜ] (as in *word*), which is a combination of both tongue and lip formation.

Very simple, childlike sounds serve as relatively good models for the vowels. As you become more familiar with the shapes, you can insist on more clearly defined vowel values. Foreign students are apt to overpronounce, just as anyone studying a foreign language might do.

AMERICAN PHONETIC SYMBOLS

Vowels

[i] he	[ɑ] spa	[ʊ] hook	[ɜ] her
[ɪ] him	[ʌ] up (stressed)	[u] hoot	
[ɛ] hen	[ə] upon (unstressed)	[e] ?bait ⎫ Pure only in	
[æ] hat	[ɔ] saw	[o] ?boat ⎭ Romance Languages	

Dipthongs

[ɑɪ] high	[ɔɪ] boy	[eɪ] hay
[ɑʊ] how	[oʊ] home	[ju] huge

Consonants

Cognates

Unvoiced	Voiced	Semivowels
Stop		[j] yes
[p] pet	[b] bet	[ɜ] red
[t] tin	[d] din	[l] let
[k] cap	[g] gap	**Nasals**
Fricative		[m] sum
[f] fat	[v] vat	[n] sun
[θ] thigh	[ś] thy	[ŋ] sung
[s] seal	[z] zeal	**Fricative**
[ʃ] rush	[ʒ] rouge	[h] he
Stop Fricative		**Rolled R**
[tʃ] cheap	[dʒ] jeep	⎰[r] (ɪt) caro
Glide		⎱(Almost exclusively
[ʍ] why	[w] we	Romance Languages)

Figure X–2. Simplified chart of American phonetic symbols. Phonetic inventory devised using Fairbanks (1960) as guide. With thanks to Timothy Monick, formerly of the Juilliard Drama Department, for checking this over.

The nearer you can come to creating the phonemes as free, independent actions, the better the articulation and the sound will be. Many of the articulation muscles have attachments to the upper surface of the hyoid bone. Because the larynx is suspended from the lower side and because there are so many interrelations of the nerves serving both the adjustments for pitch and the movements for articulation, you need to isolate each action as much as possible.

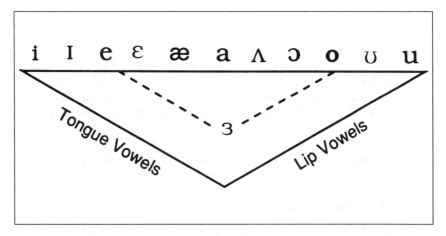

Figure X–3. The vowel triangle. This represents what are called closed vowels at each end and open vowels in the middle.

In singing, for all practical purposes there are ten pure vowels and six diphthongs. The phonemes [e] (as in *haste*) and [o] (as in *boat*) are invariably pronounced as diphthongs by Americans. This is noted in the chart. I also call your attention to the fact that, because of the prolongation of vowels in singing, the phonemes [ʌ] (as in *fun*) and [ə] (as in *upon*) become one and the same. The only advantage to using both symbols would be to indicate rhythm and stress in the flow of the language. For consistency, I am using the symbol [ə] even though it is prolonged in the exercises.

VOWEL EXERCISES

I have found these exercises to be an uncomplicated way to form vowels with a minimum of muscular involvement. The primal sound [ə] is the starting point because it only uses airflow and natural phonation. You should be well acquainted with it by now. I like to think of all vowels as having two parts, the schwa plus the shapes formed by the articulators. This is the spotlight image. Most people find the lip vowels easier, so I start with [u].

1. [u] (boot, shoe, food)
   While you prolong the schwa [ə], round your lips, much as you would if cooling a hot drink or dish of soup. You will hear the color *oo* being formed. Whisper it, [hu]. Avoid raising the back of your tongue, which would tend to decrease the resonance and produce a bottled vowel color. Let your jaw drop freely as you round your lips. Sound [hu] like a sigh.

2. [ʊ] book, hook, look
   Start by sustaining the sound you just learned, [hu]. As you prolong this sound, very slightly drop your jaw while you keep your lips rounded. It is as though you were slowly saying the word *wool*. Whisper it, [wʊ]; then sound it.

3. [o]
   Float and *boat* are considered pure by some speech scientists, as distinguished from *home* and *go*. Starting again with [hu] let your jaw drop a tiny bit further than for [ʊ]. It is like saying "whoa" to a horse, only in slow motion. Note that although I am treating this phoneme as a pure vowel, I feel Americans sound it as a diphthong [oʊ] almost exclusively. Whisper [ho], then sound it like a sigh.

4. [ɔ] hall, hawk, horn
   Begin again with [hu]. Keep your lips lightly activated but not protruded excessively. Slowly open to the word *wall*. Whisper [hɔ], then sound it.

5. [ə] hum, huff, hut
   You are now back at the starting point, jaw and lips relaxed, [hə].

We now turn to the other side of the triangle and explore tongue vowels:

6. [i] he, heap, beat
   Sustain [hə], jaw dropped passively open, tip of your tongue resting in contact with the inside of your lower front teeth. While sustaining [hə], loosely move the middle of your tongue as though saying, [həjəjəj], ending on [i]. The middle of your tongue will touch your upper teeth on each side. Avoid moving any face muscles, especially pulling back the corners of your mouth. Think of this as an isolation exercise of freely moving (wiggling) only your tongue. Lips can be slightly protruded, which

will darken the vowel color a bit toward the German [ö]. This helps to keep the back of your mouth open and the larynx resting low. Whisper [hi]; then sustain it.

7. [ɪ] hiss, him, hit

   During a freely prolonged [hi], let your tongue relax slightly from its arched position and repeat the sounds [jɪ] as in *yip*: [hijɪjɪjɪ]. Whisper [hɪ]; then sustain it.

8. [e] hate, haste, halo

   This vowel, like [o], is more often a diphthong than a pure Italian vowel. While sustaining [hi], let your tongue relax a bit more and allow your jaw to drop slightly. It is much like saying "Yea!" (or Yale). Repeat [hijejeje]. Whisper [he]; then sustain it.

9. [ɛ] head, hen, hem

   A little more relaxing of your tongue from the [hi] brings you to a sound like the word *yet*. Repeat [hijɛjɛ]. Whisper [hɛ]; then sustain it.

10. [æ] hat, have, ham

    By relaxing your jaw completely from [hi], you arrive at what Vennard (1967) calls the "nasty [æ]." His comments about the emotional connotations of this vowel sound are interesting to read. Again, starting with an easily sustained [hi] drop your jaw and tongue, saying yam. Repeat [hijæjæjæ]. Whisper [hæ]; then sustain it.

11. [ɑ] heart, hard, harm

    Because there are so many regional variations of this vowel, it is one of the most difficult for Americans to master. Try to think of how a child says "DaDa" or "MaMa." The word *father* is often used to illustrate this vowel color. Start by sustaining [hi], drop your jaw and tongue completely, sliding the sound into yah as in yard. Repeat [hijɑjɑjɑ]. Whisper [hɑ]; then sustain it.

12. [ɜ] heard, hurl, her

    This last so-called pure vowel is spelled five different ways: *or* (as in *word*), *ur* (as in *hurl*), *ir* (as in *girl*), *ear* (as in *heard*), and *er* (as in *her*). It is difficult to keep this vowel pure because of the American tendency to run it into an *r* [ɝ]. Try to avoid this fault. It is better to find this vowel by sustaining [o]. Keep your lips rounded for [o] as you let your tongue glide toward the position for [e] The result should bring you to a sound much like the ending of *lower*. It has been compared to the *eu* in

French and "ö" in German. Repeat [hoeoeoe], keeping lips rounded with only the tongue moving. The word *coerce* uses this combination of sustaining a vowel while adding another. Whisper [hɜ]; then sustain it.

DIPHTHONGS

Diphthongs are combinations of two vowel sounds, one stressed and one unstressed. It is just as important to pronounce the unstressed vowel distinctly as it is to pronounce a consonant. In the illustration of the pig, a child would see that something is missing: the tail (Figure X–4). The body of the pig is symbolic of the stressed vowel and the tail, the unstressed glide. The tail doesn't amount to much, but think how incomplete the pig looks without it.

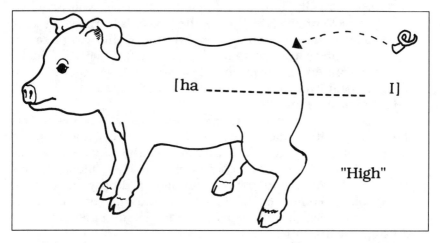

Figure X–4. Diphthong. The pig's body is symbolic of the stressed vowel, the tail of the unstressed glide.

DIPHTHONG EXERCISES

Prolong the stressed part of the following diphthongs, then glide quickly but distinctly through the unstressed part:

13. [aɪ] high   [hɑ-------ɪ]
14. [aʊ] how   [hɑ-------ʊ]
15. [ɔɪ] hoist   [ho-------ɪ]
16. [oʊ] home   [ho-------ʊ]
17. [eɪ] hay   [he-------ɪ]

In this next example, the unstressed vowel comes first. The timing is the same as for a consonant before a vowel in singing.

18. [ju] hue   [hju-------]

There are some triphthongs in English, three connected sounds that serve as a monosyllable. For example: *tire* [tɑɪɹ] or *wade* [weɪd]. If you know the stressed sound and pronounce all parts, there are no special problems.

Practice all diphthongs and triphthongs on the same exercises you use for the pure vowels.

The Prolonged Inflection Exercise

Once you have found the formation of each vowel, it may be exercised as follows:

[u] a. Sustain the word *who* and let it slide downward in an easy inflection. [hu---]

    b. Now say it slowly, as if asking a question. [hu---]. ?

    c. Speak the sound in a straightforward manner. [hu---].[1] !

When you can pronounce this sound freely, you are ready to try it on simple scales, such as in Exercise I through X of the appendix. Test all the vowels on the Prolonged Inflection Exercise before singing them on the scales. This exercise is valuable for speakers as well as singers.

---

[1]This exercise is from a book written by my great uncle, Richard Cone (1908), a master teacher of elocution who held classes at Harvard Divinity school and maintained a private studio in Boston. I vividly recall his recitations of Shakespeare. The only voice I have ever heard which reminded me of his was that of Sir Laurence Olivier.

CONSONANTS

For intelligibility, consonants are the most important elements in articulation because there are more of them, twenty-six, compared to ten vowels and six diphthongs. Consonant formations are made anterior to vowel formations. They can be thought of as releasing from their tensions back into the relaxed vowel positions.

One reason you must study and work on consonants in particular is because they have less energy in them than the vowel sounds. Every actor and public speaker learns to exaggerate or he or she will not be understood. At first you might feel self-conscious doing this, but it is important to persist.

As the movements necessary to form consonants tend to distort the purity of a relatively relaxed vowel formation, you must plan the timing of the consonant articulation so as not to infringe on the value of the preceding vowel color. I sometimes compare the consonants to doorways between rooms, which represent the vowels. You don't spend time in the doorway but its presence is very important.

Research has shown that consonants create a back pressure, which, in turn, reduces the driving force of the air and lowers pitch (Baken & Orlikoff, 1987). This seems to be an inescapable reality. Think of all consonants as having pitch, and sing through them to conceal the changes as much as possible. Let the consonant articulation be firm and crisp, dropping in and out as if the flow of the vowel continued right through. If the consonant is not imagined as sung, even though it is an unvoiced sound like s, there is an undesirable scooping or sliding of the melodic line. With good legato, no pitch change is heard, perhaps because we are so accustomed to it in our language.

The closer you come to letting these different shapes happen separately, freely, and spontaneously, the better your articulation will become. Because the larynx is suspended from the bottom side of the hyoid bone and because there are so many inter-relations of the nerves serving both the muscle adjustment for pitch and the movements of the articulators, you need to isolate each action as much as possible. Your task is similar to that of a mime artist who must isolate and control the muscles of his body and face.

Vowel sounds fall on the beat. Initial consonants, therefore, must be sounded before the beat. If this is not done, it gives the effect of a word being late and out of sync with the accompaniment. Properly executed, consonants give energy to the vowel and character to the text. It certainly adds immeasurably to the pleasure of an audience to be able to understand the words.

As shown in Figure X–2, consonants are grouped according to their characteristics. The term *cognate* refers to the fact that, in this group, each pair of phonemes is formed in exactly the same way; one is sounded by the friction of the airflow and the other, by the addition of the voice. The subdivisions on the chart, such as Stop, Fricative, and so on, are self-explanatory. The sound [w] could also be classified as a Semivowel.

Consonant Exercises

Exercises XXXIVa, b, and c in the appendix are designed to bring mobility and flexibility to your articulation. If you experience difficulty with any of the consonants, get assistance from someone who can watch and hear what you are doing.

Practice the exercises slowly at first to establish coordination. Later, you can speed up.

VOWEL MODIFICATION

It is impossible to maintain one vowel position at all pitches. Vowel modification must be mastered to facilitate a smooth transition from low to high and soft to loud. The vowels change their modal formants according to the effects of both frequency and intensity shifts. As a basic rule, the louder or higher, softer or lower a vowel is sung, the more it will migrate in color. The loudest, the highest, and lowest tones tend to be more open.

Experiments have been performed with synthesized vowels by changing the frequency at which the vowel is produced. If no components of the vowel are altered and the frequency is raised by an octave, for example, the resulting vowel value on the higher frequency is entirely unacceptable to our ears as representative of that phoneme.

A larger resonating cavity is needed to accommodate the higher frequencies and intensities in the sound waves of higher and louder tones. If this is not done, the resulting feedback can actually be a strain on the larynx. If you carried modification to an extreme, your highest notes would end up sounding very much like the schwa [ə]. This is why it is so difficult for sopranos and coloraturas to articulate distinctly in their top ranges, especially with full tones. When the muscles are loose and free, however, much more can be done with articulation.

To address this problem, Berton Coffin (1976) devised a system based on the type and range of voice, suggesting that the singer should think of the resonance of vowels in relation to the pitches being sung. For example, Coffin's charts indicate at what pitch a voice should shift from a closed [i] to a more open [ɪ] and further in an ascending scale to [e] and [ɛ]. Students have found this valuable as a guide to producing their best tones and vowel identity in going from low notes to high, or in reverse. Similar research was carried out by Ralph Appleman (1967) in his study of vowel migration. He developed an instrument called the "vowelometer" to test his results. His book, *The Science of Vocal Pedagogy*, contains a wealth of information on the scientific aspects of articulation.

My own experience with this problem has been that if you will keep thinking the vowel you want to sing, but allow the articulation positions to relax into more space for higher tones, we hear the vowel you are thinking. The larger resonating spaces needed to accommodate the higher frequencies and intensities are not necessarily produced by opening your mouth wider. In fact, stretching your mouth and bringing tension into your face and jaw can produce a countereffect and make it more difficult to sing the pitch because of the tension reflected back into the larynx. Keep the back of your mouth and throat open with face muscles relaxed. A firm, low connection with the breath is essential. It's impossible for you to hear the result the way others do. Don't try. Depend on finding an easy adjustment for the pitch. Develop your proprioception.

It is interesting to watch footage of Lily Pons as she makes her mouth opening smaller when she sings her highest notes. Of course, she is not concerned with vowel identity at that point—nor is anyone else. In fact, most high notes and great intensity are more concerned with the musical effect than with delivery of text. The voice is a musical instrument; high notes and great intensity in themselves have an emotional impact.

WORD PRODUCTION AND THE VOCAL APPARATUS

We are learning from studies with the fiberscope that far more happens in the pharynx than had been realized. We knew that the epiglottis stands up and permits a clear view of the vocal folds during pronounciation of *e* [i], or, to a degree, *ay* [e], but it had not been so obvious that a similar position is assumed while forming *oo* [u]. In fact, there is a considerable amount of interesting activity in the pharyngeal area as vowel sounds are produced (Bell Telephone Co.). That this activity appears to be involuntary is another good reason for establishing as free a condition as possible for all movements of the articulators.

The vocal folds themselves remain constant as a sound source. Present evidence indicates that there is no change at the glottis for different vowels. The voice at its source is just an uninteresting buzz. Persons with a laryngectomy have a different sound source, but can produce different vowels by changing the articulatory shapes just as others do. They learn to swallow air and time their articulation with the belching sound made in the esophagus.

In my observation, it is more profitable for singers to think of the lip vowels as "forward" and the tongue vowels as "back," even though the reverse designations are given by phoneticians. The [i] vowel, for example, has more open space at the back of your mouth than any other. That is why a doctor asks you to say [i] when he wants to look at your larynx. In pronouncing the [i] vowel in singing, the jaw must hang loosely and the lips relax.

Also, calling the [ɑ] vowel "open" is apt to be misleading. Actually, the front of your mouth needs to be open very little. It's the back of your mouth that needs space. Allow expansion in the pharyngeal area and let your larynx rest low. Having your mouth open in front, as if you were about to take a bite of something can actually result in laryngeal tension, which you definitely do not want.

To open your mouth properly requires freedom of movement in two areas. If your head was in a clamp so that you could not move it up or down, the only way you could open your mouth would be to let it drop from the hinges of your jaw. On the other hand, if your jaw was resting on a post so that you could not lower it, you would have to lift your head. In the entire animal kingdom the mouth is opened by both lifting the head (the hinge at the back of the neck) and dropping the jaw. Neither movement is excessive, but both hinges should be well oiled. It is a coordinated action.

A light glottal is often needed in English. For example, *our eyes* would become *our rise* without a glottal stop to begin *eyes*. For details on diction, I recommend two books: *The Singer's*

Manual of English Diction by Madeline Marshal (1946), and *To Sing in English* by Dorothy Uris (1971).

Actors, public speakers, and singers must learn how to "spit" out their consonants. I sometimes tell my classes, "Don't sit in the front row at a song recital unless you have brought a raincoat or an umbrella!"

The resonance center for vowels is in back of where all consonants are formed. This is another reason for a feeling that you release all consonants backwards. Maintain a "vowel alignment" by keeping a balance of resonance through all of the vowels. Maintain each vowel as long as possible to keep its purity; dismiss each consonant as cleanly as possible by bridging over the resonance from vowel to vowel. During rests, especially short ones, imagine that you continue singing. This keeps the resonance areas open so that the new phrase begins in the same space that the last one left off.

When your mouth is closed for the humming sounds [m], [n] and [ŋ], your soft palate drops down. If your palate is down for other sounds, nasality will result. In both starting the humming sounds too soon and not releasing them quickly enough, an undesirable nasality can be introduced into the vowel. For example, if the words *My nose* happened to be in the song, you would drop the [m] before [ɑɪ] and keep the beginning of the diphthong sound [ɑ] pure as long as possible. The end of the diphthong [ɪ] should not be anticipated and thus combine with the following [n], which in turn should be clearly disengaged when it is time to sing [o].

Remember that nasality and nasal resonance are two different things. Although some argue that the soft palate should be slightly relaxed in the final stages of training, it is better to keep it arched in early practice. The soft palate seems to remain arched on all vowels. This keeps the nasal port closed, except in humming, when it opens automatically. If you have a problem keeping the soft palate up, there are exercises to help in correcting this in Chapter XX on Voice Problems.

For the letter "r" as pronounced in American English, I have used the symbol [ɝ]. The rolled [r] is used in Italian and other romance languages. In some parts of the United States, [ɝ] is greatly exaggerated. The more open [ɝ] is preferred over the rolled [r] but should not be overdone.

STUDYING ARTICULATION TECHNIQUES

English has a large number of phonemes in common with German, French, and Italian. Vocally, the same techniques for articulation apply to all languages: relaxation of the extrinsic laryngeal muscles, free coordination of the articulators, and a firm connection with the breath. For the study of articulation in other languages, I recommend a special diction course for each. Books on diction can be useful. *Diction* by John Moriarty (1975) is one and *Singing in French* by Thomas Grubb (1979) is another.

Because language is employed in singing, your speaking habits can carry over. As they say, "You can get the boy out of the country, but it's hard to get the 'country' out of the boy." If your speech habits have been free and healthy, they will lead you to a healthy and uninhibited approach to singing and articulation. For the professional, it is desirable to train good habits of phonation and articulation in both speech and singing. Your progress depends on it. How well this is accomplished depends on the artist in each of you.

For examples of good articulation and diction, I would recommend listening to Dietrich Fischer-Dieskau, Elizabeth Schwarzkopf, Gerard Souzay, Eleanor Steber, John McCormick, and John Charles Thomas. Broadway singers give you every word. You may have other favorites, of course. I recommend these artists not only because of their clear pronunciation, but because of their ability to imbue the text with great feeling. After all, isn't that what it's all about?

No doubt, there will be differences in the rules for diction among authorities in every language. My goal is to help you to be understood by the simplest means possible. Please *be understood when you sing!*

Think straight. Concentrate on where you are going all the time. If you have conditioned your reflexes to respond to your thinking, you can *let* it happen automatically. And if you can do that, there should be no reason why you shouldn't *trust* your performance.

"gɔd blɛs əmɛʒˈıkə"

REFERENCES

Appleman, R. (1967). *The science of vocal pedagogy*, Bloomington, IN: Indiana University Press.

Baken, R.J., & Orlikoff, R.F. (1987). *The effect of articualtion on fundamental frequency in singers and speakers*, Journal of Voice, 1, (pp. 68–76): Raven Press.

Bell Telephone Co. (1960). *The speech chain* (film available from Haskins Laboratory, New Haven, Ct.).

Brown, O. (1953, May–June). *Principles of voice therapy as applied to teaching*, National Association of Teachers of Singing Bulletin, (pp. 16 & 21).

Coffin, B. (1976). *The sounds of singing*, Boulder, Co: Pruett.

Cone, R.W. (1908). *The speaking voice—its scientific basis in music*, Boston: Evans Music.

Fairbanks, G. (1960). *Voice and articulation drillbook*, New York: Harper.

Grubb, T. (1979). *Singing in French, a manual of French diction and French vocal repertoire*, New York: Schirmer Books.

Ladefoged, P. (1962). *Elements of acoustic phonetics*, Chicago: University of Chicago Press.

Marshall, M. (1946). *The singer's manual of English diction*, New York: G. Schirmer.

Moriarty, J. (1975). *Diction: Italian, Latin, French, German*, Boston: E.C. Schirmer.

Uris, D. (1971). *To sing in English*, New York: Boosey & Hawks.

XI

∎

PRACTICE PATTERNS

"I never practice."

This statement, made by a soloist from the Metropolitan Opera who sought my advice about a voice problem came as no surprise to me. I showed him an exercise that addressed his needs. He caught on immediately, but my hunch is that the solution seemed too easy, and that he went back to his old habit of not practicing. He didn't continue much longer at the Met, and I never saw him again.

I have worked with and observed many artists who fail simply because they fail to establish a daily routine of vocalizing. Students express amazement at discovering that the root of their difficulty was a failure to practice or to practice correctly.

Why should singing be different from any other athletic endeavor? In fact, the singer is much more fortunate than the dancer, for example, because a singer can continue to perform much later in life if he or she has taken good care of him- or herself. As Constantin Stanislavski (1972) wrote in *An Actor Prepares*, "Never begin with the results. They will appear in time as the logical outcome of what has gone before" (p. 175). Technical training frees the artist in each of you for emotional and intellectual expression.

Our study, so far, has centered on the physics of sound as applied to singing, the physiology of the larynx, and the laws of muscle growth. My objectives have been to help you do the following:

1. Discover your own voice and its potential range, size and quality

2. Condition your voice so that it responds automatically and consistently on demand
3. Sing with an effortless legato line
4. Sustain long phrases
5. Execute coloratura
6. Gain freedom of articulation
7. Maintain vocal condition
8. Avoid damage—learn the basic principals of voice therapy
9. Be your own teacher whenever you are on your own.

To quote a Chinese proverb, "Teachers open the door; you enter by yourself."

STARTING EACH DAY

No student should expect his voice to be exactly the same every day, especially when starting. You don't feel the same each morning when you get out of bed; why should your voice be just the same? Your voice is a part of your whole body. No matter how your voice behaves one day, the next morning you must start at the beginning and progress only as far as your voice will take you without strain. Be sensitive to the needs of your voice from day to day and trust your instincts. There may be times when it seems as though your voice is ready to respond without preparation. Most of the time, however, it takes slow, careful warm-ups to bring your voice to a state where it is ready to work on literature. Think of the warm-up as vocal hygiene, just as you think of washing your face and brushing your teeth each morning.

Let's state some of the principals of daily practice:

1. Take time to loosen your body to a state of release. Many people find this difficult because it isn't "singing." People seem to think that if they are going to study singing, anything that does not involve the use of the voice is a waste of time. "It is what we think we know already that often prevents us from learning" (Claude Bernard).
2. Establish body alignment and awareness of involuntary breathing. "The more you use your body sense the more developed it will become . . . . Gradually you will experience a sense of great release and deep satisfaction as your inhalations function more on their own with less help from you" (Spreads, 1978, pp. 8 & 11).

3. Think the sound and allow the airflow to do the work. Remember that your goal is to achieve the greatest freedom with the least amount of effort for the end result. The "trick is to let the body give up the inappropriate patterns without forcing it" (Ristad, 1982, p. 121).

4. Warm up the vocal muscles daily, calling on automatic pitch adjustments that are free from hyperfunction. Review Chapter IV if necessary. The great Russian pianist Anton Rubenstein is quoted as having said, "If I miss practice one day, I can tell. If I miss practice two days, my friends can tell. If I miss practice three days, my audience can tell." If the nerves are not called upon for their maxmum saturation, they will be less responsive (Sherrington, 1961).

5. Remember that each voice is different. Each singer develops at his or her own pace, independent of what anyone else is doing or has ever done. "The singing voice needs time for full development" (Brodnitz, 1953, p. 74). Good habits established early on become a foundation for all that follows. As you repeat each action, it becomes easier and easier. Soon, you will have formed habits ready to serve you as you need them.

6. Don't hurry. It takes time to develop the trust and confidence necessary to let go and let your voice show you what it can do. Keep in mind the adage, "It isn't the mountains ahead that wear you out, it's the grain of sand in your shoe." Divide your practice into several short periods rather than singing for an hour, especially at the beginning. In time, your endurance will grow, but go at your own pace.

7. Regardless of where you begin, your goal is full development, that is, to fill in those areas that are weak and missing. I compare the finished product to a circle, the ideal being optimum development of all segments within the circle (Figure XI–1). One student might begin studies with strengths in areas 12 to 2, 5 to 6, and 8 to 12; another, with strengths in areas 2 to 4, 8 to 10, and 11 to 12. In the beginning chapters of this book, I presented a series of exercises in what I believe to be a natural sequence of development. Perhaps this circle can serve as an outline to diagnose missing qualities in your voice. An accomplished artist will leave none of the segments weak enough to be noticed. Although the segments are equal in the illustration, they have varying degrees of importance.

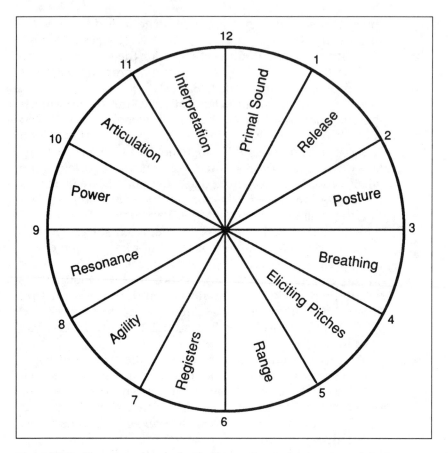

Figure XI–1. The areas of study that lead to optimum development of singing.

The technical development of your voice will continue for years. Beyond the exercises that I have provided to get you started, hundreds of scales can be found in different books. As long as you follow the principles for exercising the voice that I have outlined, there is no limit to what you can try.

LEARNING TO VOCALIZE A SONG

Many students complain that singing a song is more difficult than vocalizing. The answer to that is to *learn to vocalize the song*. In vocalizing, you have been concentrating on one element at a time. Why not approach a song in the same way? Each aspect of performing a song must be mastered in your mind. Hearing the music with your eyes, as you leaned to do in sight singing, does not mean that you can look at a song and automatically have your muscles respond to it. The elements of time, pitch, quality, tempo, intensity, articulation, meaning, mood, and musicianship must all be mastered by your mind and worked into your responses. Of course, as a solo instrument you only need to think of pitch and time. But, in another sense, you are like a conductor asking for responses from forces that you can't put your hands on.

Since you already know how to read words, I suggest that you begin mastering a song by concentrating on the musical elements. Here is one way to do it:

1. Study the rhythm. Go through the music much like a solfeggio exercise, noting and clarifying any intricate passages.
2. Now go through as if it were a study in intervals with no regard to the rhythmic patterns.
3. When these first two steps are accomplished, take a moderate metronomic tempo and go throughout the piece on "la, la, la" or some similar easy syllable, singing the notes in the rhythm. Make no attempt at dynamics.
4. Read through the words as a poem. If it is in a foreign language, translate it word by word. Attend to any diction problems before proceeding.
5. When you have mastered Step 4, read the words in the rhythm of the music. Maintain a strict tempo.
6. Now sing the words on the pitches in the rhythm, with no dynamics.
7. Thoroughly study all the expression marks, tempos, louds and softs, fasts and slows, stresses, et cetera.
8. Begin working on the song as a work of art, giving special attention to the meaning of the words and the musical phrasing.

If this procedure is carefully followed, hours will be saved in learning a song and it will be practically memorized by the time you have mastered Step 7. Most importantly, you won't have built in faulty habits due to a lack of familiarity with the music. It may seem like the long way around, but it works. Also, much of the above can be accomplished with very little demand on your vocal muscles.

WORKING ON A NEW SONG

To practice singing, especially in learning a song, it is not necessary to make any sounds at all. Think, think, think! If you have trouble remembering the words, write them out as many times as is necessary to commit them to memory. Link the end of one line with the beginning of the next in your mind. See if you can connect a chain or progression of thoughts so that one part of a song leads to the next.

Once all this has been learned, there is much to be said about getting music into your voice:

1. The melody can be sung through as a vocal exercise on any easy vowel sound. Pay no attention to dynamics at first.
2. If you find a particular section of the song vocally difficult, lift that phrase out of context and practice it as a vocal exercise, singing it a bit lower or higher until the notes come easily.
3. Next, vocalize the song on the vowels of the words only. Pay attention to where the breaths should be taken.
4. Gradually introduce the consonants, pronouncing them very lightly and loosely at first.
5. See if you are able to perform at the proper tempo and move smoothly into any tempo changes.
6. Begin to feel the true value of the consonants and where stresses need to be given. Work on this stage until all consonants have their proper value and intelligibility.
7. Now work toward the desired dynamic levels. Leave this until last to avoid strain. You should feel that you could do more if you wanted to . . . . *but don't!*
8. Present the music with a forward flow, a line, a legato. Let it move so that it expresses a continuity from beginning to end.
9. Study a piece backwards, then you know where you're going. Practice what comes at the end, perhaps the last phrase or the last page, and be sure you feel confident in singing it. Then practice the section that precedes this and carry the song to the end, continuing this process backwards to the beginning of the piece. If a particular section presents difficultly, master it before you try the whole song.

MENTAL PREPARATION COMES FIRST

Another excellent way to work on a song is to sit in a quiet room and sing it mentally. Motor coordination can be helped in this way, as well as memorization. An even better way is to memorize before the physical process is employed. There are artists who never use their voices on music until they have it completely memorized.

As you work through the song in your mind, breathe as though you were singing it aloud. Think through the music at the tempo that you will be using later. Be sure to keep the accompaniment going mentally at the same tempo in any section where the voice part has rests.

Feel the phrasing. Silently shape the words, taking care to form them loosely, maintaining the vowel positions for their time values and timing the formation of consonants as well. In your imagination, hear an inner voice singing the song. This voice is your mental image of an ideal. You will be surprised at how easily you can perform after doing this. The voice responds to the mental concept.

Think ahead. Never break your concentration by listening to yourself or thinking back about what you just did. I once had a student who was singing the tenor solos in *Elijah* with orchestra for the first time. His performance had gone remarkably well and he had one more phrase to sing. Suddenly, I held my breath because he entered half a beat late. After the performance, I asked him what happened. He said, "Gee, I was thinking, 'I've come all the way through without making a single mistake!'" A performance isn't over until it's over.

I had another student who was always dressed and ready to sing at least an hour before her appearance. During that hour she would sit quietly in her dressing room and go through the entire program in her mind. When it was time to appear, she would maintain her concentration as she walked on stage, although outwardly she greeted her fellow artists and her audience. Her performances were exemplary. As Feldenkrais wrote in 1972, "The possibility of a pause between creation of a thought pattern for any particular action and the execution of that action is the physical basis for awareness" (p. 45).

After all your mental preparation, it is time to test it out. Sing easily in your first rehearsals, either by yourself, with an accompaniment, with a conductor, or with a stage director. Let the music build to its performance level gradually. This will help to avoid instilling any habits that you do not want. A rehearsal is not a performance until you are ready to make it one. If you have been hired for the job, it is because you have the qualifications. It may not be possible to put into a rehearsal what is required for the performance. Your mind needs to absorb your relation to the elements of space plus, in the case of opera, to other performers, before it can be free for the demands of your own voice.

Each of us is born with our own set of physical, mental, and emotional qualities. These should be explored with a sense of joy and adventure, much more as play than as work. By "listening" to what your body tells you, you will know what feels right. Trust that inner sense no matter what anyone tells you!

Realize that the only competition you have is the challenge to develop your own voice to its fullest, and the challenge is to understand what the poet and the composer expressed and bring it to life through your performance.

REFERENCES

Brodnitz, F.S. (1953). *Keep your voice healthy*, New York: Harper & Brothers.

Feldenkrais, M. (1972). *Awareness through movement*, New York: Harper & Row.

Ristad, E. (1982). *A soprano on her head*, Moab, Ut: Real People Press.

Sherrington, C. (1961). *The integrative action of the nervous system*, New Haven, Ct: Yale University Press.

Speads, C. (1978). *Breathing, the ABC's*, New York: Harper & Row.

Stanislawski. C. (1972). *An actor prepares*, New York: Theatre Art Books.

XII

■

INTERPRETATION:
PROGRAM THOUGHTS

Your voice knows how to sing. It knows how to sing better than you do. Think the music and your voice will sing it for you.

Your whole body is the instrument. All it asks is that you have a thought—get out of the way—and let your sound out. Not a sound like your mother's or your father's or the latest stars in rock or opera, but your own sound, your primal sound, the sound you were born with.

By following the exercises described in the preceding chapters, you have been conditioning responses so that you can give your attention to text and musical values. By now, you should feel that singing is a natural part of you, a channel for releasing your inner feelings.

When artists have acquired their technique, they have touched base with their native selves. Since each individual is unique, the artist is able to demonstrate those qualities of his or her voice which make it different from every other voice. He uses his instrument to convey the soul and mind behind a printed page of music. Without technique, which gives the freedom to let this happen, an artist might compensate for his lack of ability, which could result in damage to his instrument.

The way to let this happen is to condition the voice to respond to mental concepts. This takes years of exacting drills and exercises, which fall into place one by one as reflexes. How did you learn to walk? You tried and failed so many times in the process that you can't possibly remember, yet you kept on trying. Once you could walk, you learned to run, to jump, to dance, and so on. If you hadn't persevered with walking, where would you be? Just as you now let your legs carry you wherever you want to go, so, by practice, you learn to let your voice perform the music according to the demands of the composer.

Music lives only when it is being performed. In singing, the real source of what can be expressed is found in the words. This is what the composer started with and what inspired the composer to heighten the meaning and emotional content with music. Many people feel that music, more than any other art form, is the language of the emotions. Singing is the most intimate form of musical expression because it is produced with a live instrument.

INTERPRETING MUSIC

Yvette Guilbert (1918), a paragon of song interpretation, said, "the requirements for a singer of song are: fantasy, originality, the power of tragic expression, literacy, culture, instinct of the plastic, sense of observation, a face with expressive eyes and mouth and an immense sensitiveness." The composer Charles Gounod told Guilbert, "Madame Yvette, for God's sake, do not take singing lessons. Your professor will kill your power of expression by giving you a 'pretty voice,' which means a 'flat' voice, and then you will be one of thousands. We have had singers with pretty, charming voices before and we shall have them again. You, yourself, have created your style; preserve it" (p. 5).

Assuming you have the vocal technique and personal traits to be an interpretive artist, it is time to develop your skills at bringing music to life.

The tools for interpretation are time, tempo, dynamics, pitch, line, diction, tone color, emotion, and meaning. As you think of the significance of these tools, how can you judge the loudness of *forte* or the softness of *piano*? How fast is *allegro* and how slow is *lento*? Do *f* and *p* mean the same thing every time you see them, even in the same song? Schumann-Heink said that you must sing out— even in pianissimos. Metronomic markings are often indicated for tempo. Yet, I have heard songs performed faster or slower than what was indicated in the score and enjoyed them very much. Think of both dynamic and tempo markings as indications of feeling. If you are sensitive to the music and the meaning of the words, you will know how fast or how loudly to sing.

Your breath capacity or the size of your voice may influence your choice of expression. One composer listening to a rehearsal for the premier of his new work put the marking *pp* in one section of the manuscript, because the artist performing the work always sang it too loudly. So what can you believe? Trust your sensibilities and know your resources so that you can recognize what is right for both you and the music. This is true musicianship.

Mahler said that no two measures are equal. Even with a score, a recurring note may require different interpretations in order to create the desired effect. For example, the opening line of the song "Daisies" by Samuel Barber reads, "In the scented bud of the morning O, when the windy grass went rippling far . . . ." (words by James Stephens), *Bud, O* and *far* are to be sung on quarter notes and the rest of the words are to be sung on eighth notes. Try reciting this with the exact same value of time and intensity on all the eighth note words. You will sound like a second grader, just learning to read. The only way to gain a sense of how the words should flow is to read them as a poem. Great song interpreters spend as much time reading the words as they do singing the music.

One great American singer was the baritone David Bispham (1857–1921). He was an advocate of singing in English for American audiences. I knew a woman who had been his accompanist, and she told me that Bispham spent more time reading a text than he did singing it. His performance of the song "Danny Deever" by Walter Damrosch, with words by Rudyard Kipling, was so vivid that Mrs. Theodore Roosevelt would only consent to his second appearance at the White House on condition that he not sing that song again. The impact of his performance had been so intense that she felt she could not experience it a second time. How many artists move an audience that much today?

PERFORMING WITH YOUR EMOTIONS

Cultivate a strong feeling for the text of any song you are to perform. Although you may have no personal experience with the emotions to be conveyed, you may know of a similar experience that will help you to identify with the words. If the song or the character you are to portray is foreign to you, you will have difficulty giving an interpretation.

There is a song with three verses, each starting with the words, "Give a man a horse he can ride . . . Give a man a boat he can sail . . . Give a man a pipe he can smoke." I once had a strapping young baritone studying with me, whose voice, I felt, would be perfect for this selection. After looking at the music for a week, he asked me if he had to learn that particular song. I said, "No," but wondered why he objected. He replied that he was allergic to horses, got seasick, and didn`t smoke! Perhaps if he were paid a thousand dollars he would have learned the song, but I doubt he would have done justice to it.

In another instance, a college junior had learned the Gretchaninoff "Lullaby" in preparation for a student recital. Though she was a lively young woman, she sang the song without emotion, as so many notes and words. I asked her if she had ever done any baby-sitting and she said that she had. Then I asked her to imagine that she was singing to a baby of her own. She paused a moment and said, "OK! Let`s sing it again." On the evening of the recital, half the mothers in the audience had tears in their eyes because of the emotion conveyed. I asked her how she had done it. "Oh," she said, "I just imagined I was holding a baby in my arms while I was singing."

Use songs that have meaning for you, songs that you like. Many times I have heard thrilling voices that left me completely cold. It's great to develop technical skill, but that`s not enough. If you want to earn a living as a singer, technical skill is just the beginning. Fortunately, there is such a range of styles, from folk and rock to grand opera, you're bound to find something that you can identify with.

A great deal of interpretative effect can be made with the proper use of consonants. Dynamic stress and the duration of consonants are powerful exercise tools. "I love you," for example, can be almost dismissed with little meaning if the *l* of love is not stressed. Or it can be imbued with great depth of feeling if the *l* is stressed and prolonged. Of course, this can be overdone. That is where artistry comes in. If a song moves quickly, then crisp, strong consonants are all the more important. "Largo al factotum," Figaro's aria in *Il Barbiere di Siviglia* by Rossini, is an illustration. The recording by Giuseppe De Luca is exemplary of the elegance and style that can be brought to this aria. A "fast" song should never be sung faster than it can be sung with clarity.

In his paper, "The Sound of Greek," W. B. Stamford (1967) quotes Dionysios of Halicannassos as having said, "The science of public oratory is, after all, a kind of musical science" and Quintillion as having said, "It is necessary that orators be familiar with both the theory and practice of music." Stamford also writes, "Poetry's earliest name in Greek primarily meant 'song' . . . . In Greek and Roman education, music and poetry were kept together in the discipline called 'mousike.' Our sentence intonation can provide a kind of melody in speech."

For expression of emotion and meaning, it would be hard to suggest a better example than Galina Vishnevskaya's (1984) recording of the "Songs and Dances of Death" by Mussorgsky. She was Russian, and having lived through the siege of St. Petersburg in the Second World War, she had seen death and dying all around her. In addition, she had the voice, technique, and musicianship to bring these songs to life.

When you listen to recordings or hear performances by great artists, notice that the accuracy of pitch as they start phrases or move from note to note is as clean as if they were playing an instrument. Some have absolute pitch, which is a great help but not essential. If you keep thinking exact pitch, that is what you get. If you do not think the pitch accurately, your voice will slip and slide and scoop.

If a piece of music is written with a time signature of 2/2 instead of 4/4, try to determine why the composer did it that way. In the song "Der Tod und das Maedchen" by Schubert, when "Der Tod" speaks, with his uncompromising message of sleep, the relentless forward march of the rhythm would be completely lost with a different time signature.

Remember that Guilbert included a face with expressive eyes and mouth in her requirements for an interpretative artist. I once read of an experiment carried out by the English throat specialists Sir Morrill Mackenzie and Sir Richard Paget in which each examined the muscle movements inside the mouth of the other as he changed facial expressions. This was done by looking through a hollow lighted tube. They detected that nature had provided us with the means of telling whether we are meeting a friend or an enemy, even in total darkness. When you change your facial expression, it alters your voice color. Try to say, "I love you," with a scowl on your face. If you turn to a dog and say, "Get out of here, you cur!" with a big smile on your face, it will probably come up and lick your hand, relying on the quality of your voice rather than the meaning of your words.

Facial expression is a marvelous tool for communication in singing. It not only gives color to the text but aids in conveying emotion. When you hear a song recital or an opera performance, you are listening with your eyes as well as with your ears.

In his book *The Expression of the Emotions in Man and Animals* (1896), Darwin quotes Muller as saying, "the conducting power of the nervous fibers increases with the frequency of their excitement." Darwin goes on to say that vocal expression is associated with different physical sensations. For example, violent outcries are associated with suffering; high pitched voice, with gentle ill treatment or light suffering; deep groans and high, piercing screams, with pain and agony.

In a 1959 article on the singing voice, Paul Moses writes, "In opera, the singer has to explore the whole personality of the role; acting is as important as singing, so the singer's concentration must be diversified and no longer completely concentrated on voice production." Moses goes on to point out that because pitch is under cortical control, this brings us close to a mental concept. Changing mental concept, therefore, means change in total concepts, the highest perfection being reached through cortical control. This sheds some light on a statement by Callas that "music is so enormous that unless you know what you're doing and why, it can envelop you in a state of perpetual anxiety and torture" (Ardoin, 1987, p. 5).

Wesley Balk (1990) discusses an experience that the actor Sir Laurence Olivier had while performing *Othello*. "Something undefinable was happening because it is something that performers cannot make happen but only be open to. Olivier is a great example because there was not an actor in the century more technically prepared with all five parts of the instrument (the mind, the emotions, the body, the face and the voice)" (p. 7).

Through thinking and practice, you can train your native sound to respond to your wishes. Concentration is essential. While performing, artists should focus so intently on what they want to express that they have no time to listen to their own performance. If they listen to their own voice, they forsake the moment to determine what will happen next.

Much depends on the performer's skill as a musician. The ability to play an instrument makes singing much easier. Marcella Sembrich was an accomplished pianist and violinist. Judith Blegen is a fine violinist. Both Sherill Milnes and Placido Domingo conduct as well as sing. Eleanor Steber entered college to major in piano before she discovered her greater asset was singing. I am told that after her retirement, Rosa Ponselle would sit at the piano and play through an entire opera, singing all the parts.

Your voice is the servant of your thoughts. Some knowledge of the mind and how it functions can be a help. In the field of sports psychology there are specialists who work with athletes to prepare them for performance. In an August 28, 1983 article from the *Sunday New York Times* entitled "Conditioning Athletes' Minds," Emily Greenspan wrote, "Practitioners teach athletes how to prepare themselves for competition without becoming too anxious or too relaxed." Do they need to be aroused or is pressure so great that they can become overstimulated? Singers are vocal athletes, so this approach applies to singers as well.

One way to build confidence is to relate new performances to successes that you have already achieved. It is like the line from an old popular song, "We did it before and we can do it again." This requires great concentration. In Greenspan's article, J. Brian Hennessy, a Stanford University graduate student in neuropsychology, explained, "Our brains do not store actual images. Sensory images are transferred into frequency patterns that are scattered throughout the brain. When we remember things, all we need is one image to reference the entire memory." That is why it helps to go through a performance mentally, thinking and hearing exactly how you want it to be, before you go on stage.

The word *color* is used to express the quality of voice that conveys meaning and emotion. I like to think of the colors in a rainbow as an illustration. Red, orange, yellow, green . . . Wait a minute. What is the color of "orange?" You can have red-orange or yellow-orange; there is no specific beginning or end. Suppose you were singing the word *home*. If you were anticipating going home as a very happy experience, the word would have a bright, happy color. On the other hand, if home had been a place of unhappy experiences and you didn't want to go back, you would sound the word with a dark, discouraging color. Conjure up an image of what you want to express and the color will be there. Emotion conveyed with primal sound gets to your gut. Although primal sound is involuntary, it can be conditioned to respond to voluntary thought.

Empathy is something else. Have you ever attended a performance where the artist was pushing and straining to get the notes, and then gone away with your throat feeling tired, even though you made not a sound during the performance? That's what empathy does. Subconsciously, your body responds and silently imitates what you are hearing. When the performance is great, you empathize with that also.

In 1979, Robert Coleman and Robert Williams reported on their study of identification of emotional states as expressed by a group of actors. The four emotions selected were joy, terror, grief, and contempt. One deduction was that the ability of the actor did not necessarily affect the average results. Another was that emotions can be correctly identified. A third finding was that *terror* elicited the fastest words-per-minute rate, followed by joy, contempt, and grief, in that order. Their conclusions could be an indication of the dynamics and tempos that might apply to a singing voice as well. It is difficult to put emotions through a laboratory test, but science seems to support empirical thinking in this area. It also seems to follow the practices that good musicians use in their singing.

UNDERSTANDING THE COMPOSER'S INTENT

To understand how a composer reacts to literature and how he would express it musically, it is of value to know something of his life and the times in which he lived. Love, for example, is a universal theme in poetry and song. Yet love is expressed differently in different cultures and in different eras. As two extremes, you could compare the music and poetry of the Classical period to that of the Romantic period. This is not to say that feelings were experienced more deeply in one period than the other. They were simply expressed in contrasting styles.

For Povla Frijsh (1881–1969), beauty of tone didn't seem to matter, as long as it expressed the song. Her voice could be rough and harsh, or it could sound as though it floated to you from the heavens. Frijsh had a great gift for language; she sang almost everything in the language it had been written. A woman who studied with her told me that in selecting new materials, Frijsh would first just read the words and live with the text for perhaps a week. If she decided she liked the words and could identify with them, she would then examine how they were treated melodically. If she felt the melody was appropriate to the words, she would then examine the colors of the accompaniment. If this pleased her after several weeks, she would learn the song. No wonder her recitals seemed to be performed exactly as the author and composer would have liked. And no wonder the audience was pleased.

In an article from the *New York Evening Sun*, William King (1940) wrote, "The best evidence of Mme. Frijsh's standing as an interpreter of songs is the large number of singers who are to be found in the audience whenever she gives a recital. To Mme. Frijsh herself, her voice is only a means to an end, and the end is letting others share her emotional response to the poetry and the music which together makes a song." In this same article Frijsh said, "If you are a real interpreter, not just a person who emits more or less pleasant sounds, your voice takes on color from a song."

Unfortunately, Povla Frijsh's recordings are difficult to find. Danish radio has featured her career in special broadcasts, so we know there are records in existence.

Another artist who followed soon after Frijsh and who picked up her reputation for being the greatest recitalist of her day was Jennie Tourel (1900–1973). We are fortunate in having a substantial number of Tourel's recordings to listen to and learn from.

PUTTING TOGETHER A PROGRAM

It was my privilege to talk with Roland Hayes (1887–1977), the son of ex-slaves and the "grandfather" of black singers in the field of classical music. Hayes told me that in putting his programs together, he would go through his music each summer to select songs for the next year's recitals. Sometimes he would take out a piece that he liked very much but feel that it was not yet settled in his voice, and put it aside. Several years later he might feel that he could do justice to this selection, but find no place where it fit in with the other music he intended to perform. Then the time would come when he had just the spot for that special piece and he would include it in his program the following year. No wonder his recitals were treasured. The last notice I saw of his appearance was when he was 83 years old! I heard him sing flawlessly at 75.

Many singers choose the same materials, but if you consider the infinite variety of voices and temperaments, you can be assured of equal variety in performance. Lotte Lehmann put her own stamp on a song in such a manner that to try to imitate her would be sacrilege. You can learn from others to the extent that you can empathize with the way a fine sound is released or the style in which the material is sung, but do not try to imitate another artist.

Do not limit yourself to singing songs in the keys in which they are published. Did the publisher or composer know you personally and put the song in just the right key for your voice? Composers may feel that a specific key best portrays the color they want to convey in their music. This should be considered if you want to transpose a selection higher or lower, but it should not prevent you from doing so. Especially when performing early music, pieces often can be transposed down because the frequency for A was considerably lower than the 440Hz we use today. Many orchestras use an even higher A than this because the conductor feels it will make the orchestra sound more brilliant. Voices don't work that way.

There has been much controversy about changing the tuning of A back to 432Hz, the standard used by Verdi. To do this, instrument factories would have to make alterations to clarinets, for example, just as they changed from the older instruments to the ones we use today. The human voice cannot be taken to a factory, however. Verdi knew well the physical limitations and potential of the voice and wrote with them in mind. It's a shame that so few conductors know the voice as a musical instrument and appreciate its potential for beauty and expression. As it is, many performers screech and strain to match the higher tuning of modern orchestras, but there must be other standards for brilliance.

Much contemporary music reflects the composer's lack of understanding of the voice and its limitations. Many composers put demands on the human voice that are unrealistic, if not, in fact, damaging. Just because some individuals are able to sing a high note once in a while does not mean that they can repeat that note over and over without allowing the muscles to rest. In one contemporary score for soprano and orchestra that I examined recently, the composer wrote high C to be sung triple forte (sometimes four fortes were written), followed immediately by triple piano, or even four or five piano markings at the same pitch! This did not occur just once, but frequently in the score, followed by two-octave leaps with extremes in dynamics being asked for on the low notes as well. In all this, the singer was also supposed to deliver text. I advised the artist who showed me this music that she could have a fine career without performing that particular work.

EVOKING THE SPIRIT OF THE LANGUAGE

Solid attention must be given to the flow of language, the stressed and unstressed syllables in the text. French relies more on time duration than on dynamic stress. The stress and flow of Italian is very different from that of German, and both differ from English. Special study is needed for each language. Meaning can be entirely changed if stress and flow are not true to the language in which a lyric is written.

Not surprisingly, many artists do best with music from their native country. What superb authenticity is brought to the performance of Spanish music by Victoria DeLos Angeles, for example. You will find the same strength in the way that Alexander Kipnis sings Russian songs.

The English oratorio school favors a rather straight tone. Early music calls for a lighter use of the voice, partly so that the voice will blend with the instruments of the day when they are used as accompaniment. You would not expect the same style in French Melodie and Italian opera. Folk songs call for yet another presentation.

Whole books have been written about interpretation and programming. I'm giving you just a peek through the door. Here is a list of books that can aid your interpretation of vocal literature:

The Interpretation of French Song, Pierre Bernac, Praeger Publications, New York, 1970.

Eighteen Song Cycles, Lotte Lehmann, Cassel & Co., London, 1945.

The Singer and His Art, Aksel Schiotz, Harper & Row, New York, 1970.

Schubert's Songs, Dietrich Fischer-Dieskau, Alfred A. Knopf, New York, 1977.

The Fischer-Dieskau Book of Lieder, Alfred A. Knopf, New York, 1977.

The Solo Song Cycle, W. D. Buckley, University Microfilms, Inc., Ann Arbor, Michigan, 1965.

An Interpretive Guide to Operatic Arias, Martial Singher, Pennsylvania State University Press, University Park and London, 1983.

Callas at Juilliard, John Ardoin, Alfred A. Knopf, New York, 1987.

The Complete Singing Actor, Wesley Balk, University of Minnesota Press, Minneapolis, Minnesota, 1977.

The New Singing Theatre, Michael Bawtree, Oxford University Press, New York, 1991.

Voice and the Actor, Cicely Berry, Macmillan, New York, 1973.

On Singing Onstage, David Craig, Schirmer Books, New York, 1978.

Stanislavski on Opera, Stanislavski and Rumyansten, Theatre Arts Books, New York, 1975.

When selecting a group of songs by more than one composer, or even the same composer, let the songs have some relationship to one another. Sometimes a single theme may be used, such as spring or flowers or love. A Brahms group could feature the nightingale. One group of songs should contrast with a following group. Who wants steak for each course of a meal? There should be meat somewhere in the program, but complement it with side dishes. A song cycle automatically determines the song order. Within a cycle, if any transpositions are considered, the key relationship must be kept in mind.

WORKING WITH YOUR AUDIENCE

One challenge of the times we live in is selling song recitals to the public. Artists need to be more human. With a few exceptions, the days when a prima donna could stand on stage and pour oceans of rich tones over an idolizing audience are over. Even these singers know they must present music that will have contemporary appeal. American audiences seem to prefer music performed in English, provided that the diction is good.

It helps to talk to your audience. Oral program notes or comments can help to create a bond between the audience and the artist. These comments need to be rehearsed, however, and presented so that they carry throughout the auditorium.

Assisting artists provide variety and interest to an evening of solo voice. There are many pleasing combinations of voice and instrument or instruments. Surprise elements add greatly to the enjoyment of a recital. A group of songs may be presented as a dramatic scene, with suggestions of acting. One artist I know put on an apron over her gown when performing "La Bonne Cuisine" by Bernstein—much to the pleasure of her audience. I once heard the cycle "Gravestones in Hancock, New Hampshire" by Nicholas Slonimsky done by two singers walking on stage as though they were walking into a cemetery and reading the inscriptions to each other. It was a great hit.

There are only a few books on program making. An excellent one, now out of print, is *The Art of Program Making* by John W. Pierce, published by E. C. Schirmer, Boston (1951). Another is the old book by Plunket Green, *Interpretation of Song*, Macmillan, London (1924). More recently, Shirley Emmons and Stanley Sontag have written *The Art of the Song Recital*, published by Schirmer Books, New York, (1979).

Personal appearance, facial expression, stage deportment, dress, stage lighting, and all the other visual accompaniments of a song recital require attention and hard work. They are all part of the art, however, and must be included. In presenting a song, nothing should be taken for granted either sociologically, psychologically, or physically.

WORKING WITH A COACH FOR INTERPRETATION

Most singing teachers can give a good start toward understanding interpretation. Many teachers are much stronger in this area than they are in vocal technique. If insufficient direction is found with a voice teacher, however, a good vocal coach should be able to give assistance. I must warn that many coaches who do not know the voice, give directions on *how* to sing a passage. Their task should be limited to indicating that a passage should be sung faster or slower, softer or louder, correcting diction, and the like. If the student does not have the technique to follow the directions of the coach, he or she may not be ready for coaching.

I've seen many unhappy results from coaches who attempted to help performers with technical problems rather than sending them back to their teachers. One young student went to not one, but three highly recommended coaches in Europe only to leave each one after a month or two and take time out to bring his voice back into condition. Unfortunately, he tried to do what these great coaches were recommending only to discover that their instructions did not agree with his voice. They tried to change his voice classification, rather than give insights into the music. Fortunately, this student had won a very prestigious competition in the United States before leaving for Europe and had the self-confidence to determine his own course.

Ultimately, you must have your own conviction about how a piece of music should be sung. Hopefully, your technique is now at the point that you are not limited in your choices. The foundation of a good performance is technique. When you have mastered vocal technique, your audience will only be aware of the steadiness and beauty of your tone. They will feel the flow of the language and not be conscious of your diction. If you perform well, your audience will be carried by the wings of your song to the highest and most noble aspirations of their own souls.

As Plato wrote, "The best music is not that which pleases most but that which satisfies the noblest. Music should hold to the principle for which it is intended . . . to imitate only that which is good, noble and dignified. Bad music is more dangerous than anything else as with its pleasing powers it may teach bad morals."

THE BEAUTY OF LIVE PERFORMANCE

It is impossible to equate the technique required for live performance with the techniques employed by a singer using a microphone. Many popular recording artists would be lost in a concert hall without amplification. Barbra Streisand and Connie Francis achieved fame and riches that would have been impossible a hundred years ago. On the other hand, they have developed techniques that are the stock and trade of popular recording artists, skills that a classical singer could not duplicate. Popular and classical singers live in different worlds. They have instruments that are physically different and they use different vocal techniques. In spite of these differences, the same rules for healthy voice use apply to each.

Fortunately, recordings have preserved performances from the beginning of the twentieth century. We can only guess at what singers sounded like before then, and even for the artists whose recordings we do have, our ability to grasp their talent and contributions is limited by the crude recording equipment available in their day. Add to this the fact that not all artists recorded well.

Even today, technicians sitting at the control table can alter what comes through to them according to their own standards. If you want to know what an artist sounds like, you must hear the artist in person. I can bear witness to this fact by comparing excellent recordings of Rosa Ponselle to my experience of hearing her at the old Met in New York. The singers performing before her entrance were so good that I couldn't imagine how she could be any better. But when she started to sing, I had the peculiar sensation that everyone else on the stage had suddenly shrunk. It was as though I was seeing them through the wrong end of my opera glasses. Without being overpowering, Ponselle's voice enveloped you like a tidal wave of warm tone. Two other voices, in my experience, have had a comparable affect: Kirsten Flagstad and Montserrat Caballe, each with her own unique quality. As great as the recordings of these artists are, nothing compares to hearing them in person.

To quote Nellie Melba (1922) once again,

Always treat words and music with respect, for they are not yours. You are merely the vehicle for presenting them to the audience.

Show respect to the "Poet" 1) by studying the words until the very heart of them is yours; 2) by enunciating the words clearly so that the audience may understand them easily; 3) by pronouncing the words correctly, so that educated ears may not be irritated; 4) by giving to the words the natural inflection and accent, so that the emotion they express is conveyed to the audience.

Show respect to the "Composer" 1) by singing what he has written, down to the last double dotted demisemiquaver; 2) by paying attention to, and carrying out, all marks of expression; 3) by studying the shape of each phrase and by handling your voice so as to bring out that shape; 4) by studying the relation of each phrase to the whole.

The eternal task of song can never be finished in a single lifetime. That is the beauty and fascination of the art.

THINK LET TRUST!

REFERENCES

Ardoin, John (1987). *Callas at Juilliard*, New York: Knopf (p. 5).

Balk, W. (1990, August). [Interview], *New York Opera Newsletter*, 3, (8), (p. 7).

Colman, R. & Williams, R. (1979). *Identification of emotional states using perceptual and acoustic analysis*, Transcripts of the 8th Symposium, Part I, New York: The Voice Foundation.

Darwin, C.R. (1896). *The expression of the emotions in man and animals*, New York: Appleton.

Greenspan, E. (1983, August 28). *Conditioning athletes' minds*, The New York Times.

Guilbert, Y. (1918). *How to sing a song*, New York: Macmillan.

King, W. (1940-April 13). [Article]. *Music and Musicians*, New York Evening Sun.

Melba, N. (1922). *The Melba method*, [Article], London: Chappell.

Moses, P.J. (1959, May). *Pathology and therapy of the singing voice*, Archives of Otolaryngology, 69.

Stamford, W.B. (1967). *The sound of Greek*, Part II, Speech and Music, Berkeley, Ca: University of California Press.

Visnevkaya, G. (1984). *Galina, a Russian story*, San Diego, Ca: Harcourt Brace.

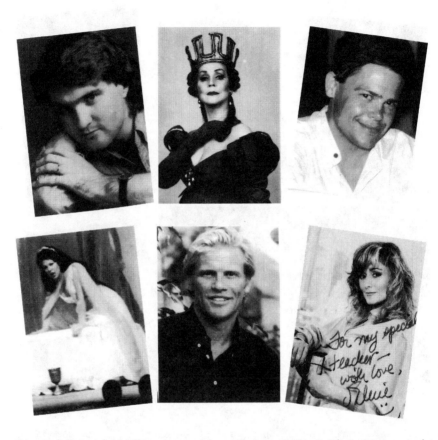

(Upper, left to right) William Joyner (photo Christian Steiner), Olivia Stapp as Lady Macbeth in *Macbeth* (courtesy Metropolitan Opera), Gregory Lorenz. (Lower) Sandra Walker as Lucretia in *The Rape of Lucretia* (Spoleto Festival); Bo Skovhus, Valerie Wilson.

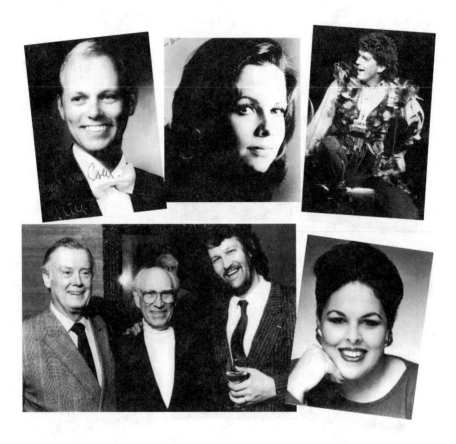

(Upper, left to right) Peter Grönlund, Judith Blegen, Sten Byriel as Papageno in *Die Zauberflote* (Danish Royal Opera). (Lower) James King, Oren L. Brown, and Poul Elming (photo Peter Schaaf), Theresa Santiago.

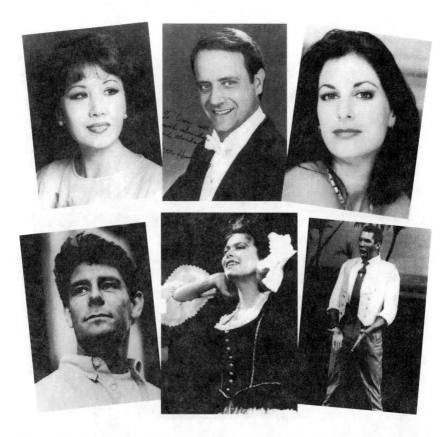

(Upper, left to right) Kang, Mi Ja, Jon Humphrey, Madelyn Reneé. (Lower) Claus Dam as Valentino in *Kiss of the Spiderwoman*, Djina Mai-Mai as Zerbinetta in *Ariadne auf Naxos* (Danish Royal Opera), Ben Holt as Sportin Life in *Porgy and Bess* (courtesy Metropolitan Opera).

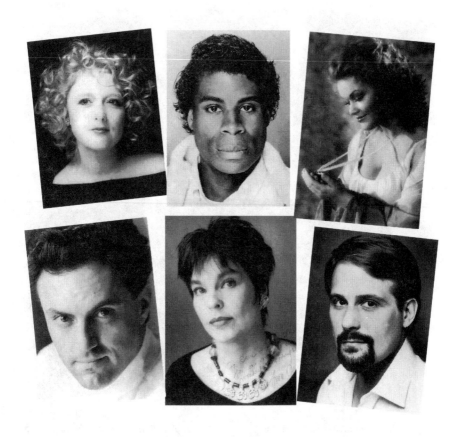

(Upper, left to right) Sofie Ottosen, Brian Matthews, Eva Johansson as Fiordiligi in *Cosi fan tutti,* (Vienna Stateopera). (Lower) Frank Lopardo, Anne Lisa Berntsen, John Thade.

XIII

■

REQUIREMENTS FOR A PROFESSIONAL CAREER

Whatever happened to Mary? . . . Tom? . . . Betty? . . . They had such wonderful voices. I thought their names would be in bright lights long before this. Do you remember how Mary brought the house down when she sang for Pavarotti in that master class at Juilliard? All he could say was, "Please, sing it again for me, just the way you did it." I heard that managers were after her to sign her up. Whatever happened?

Thousands enter colleges and conservatories every year to study singing. Many have stars in their eyes. But when experienced teachers audition the young aspirants, they know before they have heard five notes whether they are interested in hearing the rest of the piece or not. Of course, out of courtesy they listen to two or three selections. Auditioning for a Broadway show might be quite different. You sing the last sixteen bars of a number and, if you're lucky, they ask what else you have with you. But, more often than not, it's, "Thank you. Don't call us. We'll call you."

Let's assume that you have proved your talent. You have finished your academic studies and have sung leading roles in several productions. You have even been paid to sing outside of school several times. Let's go further. A management has given you a one-year contract and you have already fulfilled several engagements. Are you through learning? Are you really on your way? What else is there to do?

I knew an exceptionally talented young bass-baritone who had been hired to join with three others to sing excerpts from different operas on a radio program, under the direction of a conductor from the Metropolitan Opera. A year later I met this man's brother on the street and asked what had happened to my talented friend.

"How well did you know him?" his brother asked. I told him that I knew him quite well. We had sung together in several ensembles. "Then you know how he loved to liven up a rehearsal by cracking jokes. In New York, he couldn't keep his mouth shut and the conductor found him objectionable."

So that was it. He was a very bright young man, always well prepared, and rehearsals got boring. He might have gotten away with his antics one or two times, but serious musicians can't work with someone who lacks discipline, and apparently he was invited out.

A sense of humor can be a saving grace in many situations. Often, a light touch can clear the air when the atmosphere seems threatening. Clear heads can function much better if animosities are avoided and a friendly attitude prevails.

WHAT IT TAKES TO GO PROFESSIONAL

It is difficult to think of a career that requires a greater variety of skills or a longer period of hard work and discipline than that of a professional singer. The rewards are great to those who succeed, but considerable skill and maturity are required.

How are you going to know what you can do unless you try? A teacher can help pinpoint strengths or weakness, but teachers are not omniscient. A number of very famous singers were told early in their careers that they had no talent and were wasting their time. I have had some students who seemed to have great promise who never accomplished anything of importance, and others who worked very hard and developed into first-rate artists. This is what makes teaching so interesting.

A teacher cannot have a career for his student—he cannot keep pushing and wishing that the student will become what might have been if he were in the student's place. The student must possess that inner drive him- or herself. Let me pass on to you an inspiring incident that was related to me when I was in high school.

I studied piano with a man who came to my hometown from Boston every weekend to teach and direct music in one of the city's churches. He traveled by train. One busy weekend, he walked from car to car trying to find a seat. A very elegantly dressed lady who was alone asked him if he would care to share her seat. Hesitantly, he accepted. She immediately started a conversation. To his surprise, she said, "You're Mr. Eaton, aren't you?"

"Yes," he answered.

"You don't know me, but I know your mother, and I thought it was you. Are you still teaching music?"

Very much mystified, he said that he was.

"Then perhaps this story will interest you," the lady went on. "Many years ago a talented, good looking young girl with plenty of money went to a famous teacher in Boston to study singing. Everyone thought she would become a great star. At the same time, a plain young lady who had very little money went to the same teacher and was turned away. She insisted that the teacher give her a chance, and he did so reluctantly. The young lady worked very, very hard. It took her twice as long to learn many things as it did some of the other students." She paused. "You seem very puzzled, Mr. Eaton."

"I must confess, I am," he answered.

"Well, I'll not keep you in suspense. I am the young lady whom everyone thought would become so great, and neither you nor anyone else on this train knows who I am. The plain little girl who had to work so hard is Mme. Lillian Nordica."

Nordica (1857–1914) was the first great American "Isolde" and "Brunnhilde," the first American to sing at Bayreuth. She had such a great voice and fine training that she could sing "Brunnhilde" one night and "Violetta" the next. Her book, *Hints to Singers*, was transcribed by William Armstrong (1923) after her untimely death while on a world tour. I call her book the common sense guide to singing and consider it one of the most helpful and inspiring books ever written for students. Her birthplace in Farmington, Maine, has been preserved as a public shrine.

"It Takes More Than Talent to Build a Musical Career," was the headline of a 1984 article by Bernard Holland for *The New York Times*. He quotes an anonymous manger as saying, "I thought that talent counted for half in the making of a successful career. Now I think it may only count twenty percent" (p. 1).

A thought-provoking and instructive address was given by the late Joseph Lippman at a convention of the National Association of the Teachers of Singing some years ago. I dedicate this chapter to his memory. In this address, Lippman gave the following requirements in summary of a discussion among a group of managers who were trying to clarify the factors that brought success and prevented success among vocal artists:

1. *Voice:* Obviously something a singer must be endowed with in generous quality and proportion. It is one thing to be admired in your home surroundings, but quite another to measure up to the standards required to earn a living. In classical singing, a voice should be able to hold its own as soloist with an orchestra or large choral group. Rare are those who find enough work as recital artists to support themselves as recitalists. Not only that, but in today's market you do not have the opportunity to be paid substantially for recitals unless you have already earned your laurels in opera or other large-scale works.

2. *Technique:* the means to the end. It is a skill that can be learned. Good health is a very important factor toward optimum development.

   If you have not taken the time to develop your technique, you fall into the danger of making your voice respond, which can lead to hyperfunction. Hyperfunction is one of the most common causes of vocal malfunction.

3. *Flair and Poise:* the earmarks of self-confidence, are represented by a spark of responsiveness, individuality, and "daring-do." These qualities are inborn for the most part.

4. *Interpretive Ability:* calls for many things, but especially a strong imagination and the ability to project a story. Great interpreters have the skill to identify with text or, in the case of opera, with the characters. This skill can be learned, but aptitudes vary.

5. *Musicianship and Musicality:* interrelated, yet different. Musicianship is a craft that can be studied and learned through solfeggio, harmony, and counterpoint. Musicality, on the other hand, is that innate sense of how a piece of music should be performed. It is a true mark of artistic skill and you almost have to be born with it. Listen to the nuances brought into play by such artists as Alexander Kipnis or Richard Tauber.

6. *Physical Appearance:* can be greatly enhanced by taste in clothes as well as by good posture, bearing, and deportment. A beautician can do wonders for a person who might be considered plain. I have known performers whose physical handicaps were overlooked by the audience because of the way they carried themselves, and because they had a great deal going for them in every other way.

Having fine features is not necessarily the basis for good appearance, but weight problems have kept many promising vocalists from being engaged. Managers know that audiences want to be pleased by what they see as well as by what they hear.

When Flagstad began her great Wagnerian career, she had an admirable appearance. Videos of Callas suggest that her voice was not adversely affected by her slimming down to an agreeable figure. If you have a problem with weight and really want to do something about it, consult a doctor. Calorie counters are also very instructive. It takes will power!

7. *Stage Personality:* self-confidence that conveys to the audience, "I belong here." It is not ham, and it is not showoff, although elements of both may be present. The controlling factor is good taste, a sense of proportion, giving the impression that you are not at all aware of the audience at the same time that you are very much aware of holding their attention with everything you do. It is an art that can be improved through study, but there has to be a good foundation to work on.

8. *Ability to Handle People On and Off Stage:* a tall order, but most important. It is a sense of being part of a team working together for mutual benefit. Tact, modesty, moderation, and authority are all intertwined in this relationship. A strong feeling that everyone is a friend communicates the kind of cooperation that would help to develop this very necessary attribute in an artist. Assistance can come from the least expected sources.

9. *Basic Repertoire:* can be acquired. To qualify as a professional, you must be ready to step in on short notice to perform music that belongs to your voice category. There are many stories of singers contacted at the last minute to fill in for others. A basic repertoire is essential if you expect to have management. How can management find engagements for a lyric soprano who doesn't know something akin to Micaela in *Carmen* or the Mozart *Requiem*, for example? Six to eight opera roles and as many oratorios or cantatas are a minimum.

10. *Reliability and Dependability:* have both kept many artists busy while others with seemingly greater talent stood by. Prima donnas who miss rehearsals or arrive late are no guideline to success.

Rehearsals require patience. Many people are involved. Attention cannot be given to one individual seeking to do his part and leave early. Being alert and thoroughly prepared are marks of professionalism. Nothing is more exasperating to a director than having to hunt down an artist when his or her cue comes along, or to watch him or her fumble through material at the last minute.

It is also essential to keep appointments and to be prompt when working with teachers and coaches.

11. *Experience:* not the exclusive domain of professionals. There are opportunities everywhere for those willing to pursue them. Parts of a recital can be given for all sorts of institutions seeking entertainment. These include schools, hospitals, homes for the elderly, churches and other nonprofit organizations. The confidence gained in standing up before such groups and winning them over is invaluable. Summer programs in opera, school productions, and community-based amateur groups are good testing grounds as well. Think of these engagements as an opportunity to test the skill and materials you hope to bring to market.

12. *Love for the Art:* A compulsion to sing is so important that if it's not there, daydreams of professional success are just that—daydreams. The drive, the ambition to succeed are the spark plugs that make the motor go in spite of disappointments and setbacks. And don't believe for a moment that the road to success is lined with roses. If there are problems, face them and do something about them. No one is right all the time. Making mistakes and then picking yourself up to carry on is part of learning. Your love of singing must give you the courage to say, "OK, let's try it again!"

13. *Physical and Emotional Health:* almost as important as having an outstanding voice in the first place. Predisposition to colds or allergies can not only harm performances but can cause them to be canceled, giving the performer a reputation for unreliability. Artists can't have confidence in themselves if their health is not robust. They will be tempted to compensate and thereby develop bad habits. Poor emotional health can lead to wrong relations or misunderstandings with fellow artists, managers, and others.

14. *Efficient Management and Publicity:* can make the difference between having opportunities to be heard and not. Management can notify you of auditions. Publicity can help attract the audience. Good management will help you develop your strengths and correct your weaknesses. The artist must produce the goods, however. It is often said that management is not interested in an artist until he or she has developed such a reputation that management is no longer needed. Obviously, this is not true. The point is that management must

have something tangible to sell. Good management can free you of the job of selling yourself. Confidence is necessary on both sides.

15. *Timing:* a factor you can control. If you are not ready to perform a work, you should not accept an offer, even if you fear you will never get another chance. To do otherwise would be a disservice to yourself and to your management. Stick to the music that you know and feel good about and hope for the best. An opportunity is not an opportunity if you are not prepared to make a thoroughly professional appearance. Timing can make you or break you. Marilyn Horne developed her skills for many years before she accepted an offer to appear at the Met.

These fifteen points shed much light on the kinds of training, preparation, and experience that are necessary for professional success. It is also a great help to have family relationships which support your ambition. There is enough hell to face from the competition without having to contend with it at home as well.

Many young musicians fail to look at the professional field from a business standpoint. What is the market? How many singers are earning 100% of their livelihood with their voices? In an April 1980 article in *Fugue*, the distinguished manager Harold Shaw stated, "A ten to fifteen year waiting period is not a long time for an agency to observe a performer before approaching him or her to join a major management. It is also not unusual for an artist to join one of the smaller managements and change to a major management later on."

LEARNING TO AUDITION

In starting a career, auditioning is the name of the game. A very successful Broadway singer once came for his lesson all dressed up, even though it was still morning. "You look as if you were going somewhere," I said. "No, I've already been. I've just had two auditions," he answered. "I manage to get some kind of work in one of every twenty-five auditions. Many of my friends who also live from their singing get one job out of about every fifty auditions."

That's the way it is in Broadway and commercial singing. And it isn't always the best talent that gets the job. I had a student who auditioned for the Muni Opera, the summer musical program in St. Louis. I was actually very surprised that he got in, and I think he was, too. When I asked him about the audition, he told me that three singers had been chosen before him, but none of them could be at the opening rehearsal, so he won by default. Edwin McArthur, musical director of the Muni Opera for many years, had these suggestions regarding auditions:

1. Select songs to show your voice.
2. The verse is *never* better than the refrain.
3. Pick the section of the song that shows you best.
4. Sopranos, show your high voice; altos, show warmth.
5. If you do a "cut" version, announce it.
6. Do not carry anything with you that you do not wish to sing.
7. Avoid songs that you know are sung often and done well.

A student once told me that she had, at last, learned how to audition. She said she would walk on stage filled with a feeling of love for singing and confident that she could technically express what the music required. She only brought music that she could identify with. She held the thought that she wanted to share what she was feeling with her listeners. She put all thought of being criticized out of her mind. Instead, she held the thought that she would present herself in the best manner that she knew how. The judges would either like her or not. That was their problem. With this frame of mind, I believe that this student had learned not only how to audition, but also how to perform.

In a feature article about bass Samuel Ramey and his start at the New York City Opera, it was reported that he had his first audition as a result of writing a note personally, since he did not have management. After the audition, he heard nothing for several months. Then he received a request to sing for the judges on stage. Again, no word was received for some time. One morning a call came for him to sing for Julius Rudel at 1:00 that day. It was fourteen months after his initial letter that he made his debut as Zuniga in *Carmen*.

PERFORMING FOR THE LOVE OF IT

Why do people study singing? I believe that the common denominator is that they like to sing. Study satisfies a personal need for self-expression and inner fulfillment. The difficulty is that students, and their teachers, often cannot tell what lies ahead until they have traveled together for a period of time. I do not believe in falsely encouraging anyone. Students need to face reality, to test themselves against the standards of the profession, and to discover who they are as individuals. There might be tears, but it is better to shed them sooner than later. Life is not easy, but is made no easier by avoiding the truth.

To quote Lilian Nordica, "If one has the voice that warrants a career, nothing can keep one from the operatic stage; if one has not the voice, nothing can put one there. Great discipline, from early years, is required of all who would become professional singers, but it is the loveliest life in the world" (Armstrong, 1923, p. 167).

Is the kind of life required of a star performer the way you want to live? It can be a lonely existence. I have known young singers with great talent who wanted more settled lives than they could hope for as professionals. They have found happiness and are at peace with themselves. Some have found work in fields connected with music, such as managing, teaching, and radio announcing.

Baryshnikov, the great dancer and choreographer, was quoted in the Sunday *New York Times* of May 16, 1982 as saying, "If I am stern, it is because I put myself in the dancer's place. When young dancers are technically ready, they still need ego and mental stamina to cope with the pressures of audiences, bad reviews and tough conversations with myself. A good dancer must have guts and discipline." This is good advice for all public performers.

The greatest artists never stop studying and analyzing their own performances to find ways to improve. The actress Cornelia Otis Skinner grew up in a theatrical family, her father being the great Shakespearean actor Otis Skinner. Ms. Skinner had nearly finished the long run of a play on Broadway. At the end of the next to the last night's performance she asked a fellow actor to stay for a few moments to see if they couldn't improve a detail in one of their scenes. This is the kind of dedication that marks a true professional.

To summarize, you must be endowed with great native talent. Nothing can take its place. That talent must be developed if you are to reach your potential. The time it takes will vary from individual to individual since no one else is exactly like you. You must build on your greatest strength but keep the whole picture in mind so that no weaknesses will keep you from the success you deserve.

REFERENCES

Armstrong, W. (1923). *Lillian Nordica's hints to singers*, New York: Dalton, (p. 167).

Baryshnikov (1982, May 16). [Interview], *The New York Times.*

Holland, B. (1984, Feb. 19). It takes more than talent to build a musical career. *The New York Times:* Arts & Leisure Section, (p. 1).

Shaw, H. (1980, April). It takes more than virtuosity to build a career. *Fugue* magazine, (p. 54).

XIV

■

CHORAL SINGING

There are many levels of choral groups. Some large churches have five, six, or seven choruses, ranging from the "cherubs" (children not over 6 or 7 years old) to the "chancel choir" (primarily adult members, some as old as 60 or 70). Public schools typically have three choruses: elementary, and junior and senior high. Colleges may have freshmen choruses, separate choruses for men and women, early music ensembles, opera groups, and university chorales. Then there are community choruses and, of course, professional groups such as the Robert Shaw Chorale, famous for many years. There are Broadway show choruses, professional opera choruses, and many professional groups with distinct styles and repertoires.

One thing all choruses have in common is the use of the human voice as a musical instrument. Good choral conductors know the range and dynamic possibilities of the instruments they direct. The difference between voices and musical instruments is that voices don't come from factories. In fact, choral conductors shape and build vocal instruments by the very way they give instruction. They act as a singing teacher to the extent that many voices under their direction have never had private lessons.

Every voice has a unique quality, so each choral group will have a unique sound, depending on the combination of voices brought together. As participants change from year to year, there will be changes in the overall quality of the ensemble.

One means of securing the sound wanted, and preserving continuity, is through auditions. Depending on the size of the community in which he or she works a choral director may have a greater or lesser pool of talent to choose from. In smaller communities, this may mean having a two-part choir for a year or two, rather than a three- or four-part group. If that's the case, don't be discouraged. There is a wealth of material for two-part choirs, as well as unison, descant, and polyphonic music. A strong two-part choir is better than a weak three- or four-part choir.

SELECTING VOICES FOR A CHOIR

Where there is an ample supply of talent to choose from, one of the points to keep in mind when selecting singers is voice size. While it is good for someone with a big voice to learn to sing softly, that voice should not be "held down." Without the right understanding of voice production, such a person might tend to hold in or squeeze his voice. Often a singer with a big voice can be given special instruction and serve as a soloist as well as a valued member of the group. Some choral conductors select a voice from each section and offer private lessons, thus providing the choir with soloists.

Selecting voices for a choir should always be done from the standpoint of doing what is best for each individual. If this is not followed, voices will not contribute their best abilities and the ensemble will not be able to produce its best results. Because strengths and weaknesses in young voices change from year to year in the make-up of high school choirs, it is often desirable to select the music for the coming year after the new group has been formed. High school voices should be retested at mid-year to find out whether or not they need to be moved to a different section. You can always find new music if necessary, but you cannot replace a voice that has been damaged by singing in the wrong tessitura.

A high school freshman came to me for study. I thought she had been studying singing for some time, but doing the wrong things. It turned out that she had never taken lessons, but in the eighth grade choir she was told to "sing out" on the soprano part so that the other students could follow her. She was a good musician, but she was not a soprano! We found she was a mezzo and, because she was changing schools, she could now join the altos. When she finished high school, she applied for admission to a music school and was admitted and granted a scholarship—as a mezzo.

A young man who had an easy high range as well as a rather low extension was told that he should be a bass. He found that his throat got tired "making enough sound" on those low notes. Fortunately, he hadn't done this long and, as he started study, he understood that what was easiest was best for his voice, so a tenor was saved—a beautiful one with no break into the high range. It was simply that, at seventeen, his upper notes had never had much exercise and therefore had no chance to grow. I could cite many more cases like this. The reader may wish to refer to Chapter VI on Voice Classification and Children's Voices.

EXERCISING THE VOICE PROPERLY

A choral director should devote the first ten or fifteen minutes of each rehearsal to voice warm-up. In the first rehearsals of each season, even more time could be spent, as this discipline saves time later on. The exercises for a group are the same as the exercises given in Chapters I through V, with voices singing in unison. High voices should sing low notes more softly than low voices and vice-versa.

Encourage teenagers and young adults to especially exercise the Register 3 (falsetto) part of the voice. This should be done lightly, with the larynx resting in a low, relaxed position, but never pulled down.

Junior high boys or even senior high and male college freshmen might object at first. There can be the same problems of voices "breaking" as there would be for a solo voice. Follow the directions given in Chapter V to correct this difficulty. Although some young men think of this as "sissyish," I remember one high school conductor who had no trouble getting the fellows to vocalize in this manner. He was also the wrestling coach!

Choirs that follow this routine will have no difficulty later on with a shortage of tenors. It also follows with girls' voices that, with proper vocalizing and learning how to get into the Register 2 (chest) voice, there will be enough altos as well as first sopranos.

Many people do not realize that a musical instrument responds better after being used. If an instrument has been in storage, several days or weeks of use may be required before it responds with the best quality. If the woodwinds, brasses, and strings are improved by being warmed up, think of how much more this applies to the muscles, tissues, and nerves of a singer.

Muscles reach peak efficiency after a period of twenty or thirty minutes of use. Athletes get their blood circulating and their nerves reaching into every available fiber before a competition by warming up. When muscles have been prepared, they can perform for a relatively long period of time before fatigue sets in. With short breaks, this could encompass a one- or two-hour period. In professional groups, a second two-hour period is possible, provided the rehearsal is well paced.

Many choral directors are so anxious to hear the finished piece that they fail to attend to the many details necessary for a successful choral production. Voices may be stressed and damaged as a result. Unfortunately, this is true in professional groups as well as high shool, church, and other amateur ensembles. Voices may be rehearsed too long or pressured to sustain unhealthy volumes.

WORKING WITH THE LEVEL OF THE GROUP

In selecting music for a group, the vocal level of the group must be kept in mind, "The Anvil Chorus" from Verdi's *Il Trovatore* would hardly be appropriate for a high school choir. The same care should be taken in finding material for choirs as would be applied in selecting material for a solo voice.

There is nothing in choral singing that doesn't have to be learned in the brain first. As in all other singing, a choral member's voice responds to a mental concept. Much valuable time is wasted trying to sing through music that is unfamiliar. Few choral groups are so good at sight reading that they would not benefit from taking the music apart.

As described in Chapter XI on Practice Patterns, a choir can go through a composition sounding the rhythms, with no pitches. If this is done staccato, with just a quick "Da" for each new note, anyone who is not getting the rhythms correctly will stick out like a sore thumb. Following a similar pattern of just singing pitches staccato will also expose any wrong notes very quickly. All of this can be accomplished without undue wear and tear on the voice.

When words are introduced, reading them first in the rhythm of the music gives an opportunity to correct pronunciation and to time consonants. Attention can also be given to timing consonant values within a legato line. This is a particularly beneficial way of practicing contrapuntal music.

You may wish to review Chapter X on Articulation. What I say there applies as much to choral singing as it does to the solo voice. The analogy I make in that chapter between colors of the rainbow and vowel colors could be helpful in getting a blend of vowel tone without undue facial contortions. Lyrics with a solemn message would be sung with darker vowel values, for example. Identifying with meaning is as important for a group as it is for a soloist and will help bring depth of feeling to the text.

If a particular section is having difficulties, their problems may be worked out in a section rehearsal. But if the entire chorus is assembled, the other parts can hum their music while the section having trouble is singing. Strong singers can be asked to rest while the others are solving problems. A choir will be only as good as its weakest member. Asking certain members of a choral group to "lead" their section can be damaging to them and undermine efforts to achieve a well-balanced choral tone.

If you allow members of the choir to sit during rehearsals, have them sit away from the backs of their chairs. Although it might seem as though this requires more effort, I find singers do not get as tired sitting this way. Members should hold their music away from their bodies; this helps keep the rib cage expanded and the conductor in view.

With amateur and school groups, members should be encouraged to use their voices on days when they do not have rehearsals. They can practice the individual parts or try some of the warm-up exercises on their own each morning. Singing two or three times a week is good, but five or six times a week is better.

When learning new music, sing it through on a single vowel or hum it. The intervals and harmonic combinations can be worked out much better this way. Do not try to tackle words, rhythms, pitches, tempos, and dynamics all at once. It is also better to learn new music singing softly, and on the slow side. This saves wear and tear on the voice and avoids forming incorrect vowel responses.

Most choral singers use their voices much more loudly than is necessary. They are competing with surrounding voices—trying to hear and assure themselves that they are on the right notes. One antidote is to have choral singers use cotton in their ears once in a while. Singing correctly, chorus members may not hear their own voice at all. Feeling the sounds inside is all the assurance they need. Relying on feeling rather than sound reduces fatigue and gives a keener sense of floating on the choral tone.

Conductors, as an experiment: Divide your chorus into two equal parts. Have section "A" sing a short passage the way they ordinarily would, and let section "B" listen. Then have section "A" repeat the passage, thinking it just the same way, but with their fingers in their ears. Repeat the experiment with section "B" singing and section "A" listening. This will demonstrate how much choral singers tend to change their voices because of the sounds around them. If singers can learn to feel what they are doing rather than listen for it, the blend and quality of the group will be greatly enhanced, and the singers themselves will find they are less tired.

A choral director can often achieve the kind of tone color wanted by placing singers in specific relation to each other. The following illustration (Figure XIV–1) is a simplification of what could be carried out with a larger group. Take any three singers in a section and have them sing in unison, placing them first as in Position Number 1, then Position 2, and so forth.

B		C		A	B	A		A	
1) A	C	2) A	B	3)	C	4) B	C	5) C	B, etc.

Figure XIV–1. Voice Blending Experiment

The combined quality will vary with each of these changes, but, hopefully, one of these will be close to what the director is looking for. By placing the voices in varying positions in a larger group, different qualities will also be noted. Finally, an exact location will be found for each voice to produce the optimum desired blend.

Ideally, each singer would use his or her voice in the same manner, no matter where he or she was standing. In fact, however, singers naturally adjust their voices to the sounds they hear around them. When I have exercised voices in a choral group over a period of six to eight rehearsals, the resulting tone mass is relatively satisfying, regardless of where the singers are placed.

With college choruses, if there are students in the ensemble who are studying privately, it is important that the choral conductor stick to basic principles concerning voice use. A student experiencing voice problems probably should not be taking part in group singing until he or she is headed in the right direction. If choir work is part of the degree requirement, a consultation between conductor and voice teacher may be helpful. Experimenting with the right positioning, as in the examples I've given above, can often help in such a situation.

Another "game" useful for discovering how well each section of a choir knows its part is to have all the sections follow and think their music, but to have only one section sing at a time. This section can stop and another continue without interrupting the music whenever the director wishes. Believe me, each section will be eager to demonstrate that it really knows the music if this is done—and, again, it saves wear and tear on the voice.

Thinking through the meaning of text and the musical values before actually putting them together works every bit as well for a choir as for a solo voice. I have discussed these techniques in Chapters XI and XII on Practice Patterns and Interpretation.

THE CHORAL DIRECTOR

If choral directors are working for the same objectives that a private teacher is working for—free production, good voice color, concentration of tone with equal vowel balance, vowel modification for high and low tones, loud and soft singing, automatic pitch adjustment (i.e., thinking the pitch and letting the airflow do the work), good posture with easy low breathing, free and easy but clean and crisp articulation, understanding the text so that meaning and emotions are reflected in the tonal color, a sense of legato line within a harmonic balance—singing in a choir should not be injurious to a voice.

If a choral conductor does not have a good ear for the potentials of the human voice, he or she is working with the wrong musical instruments. I have known choral conductors who could hardly sing a note to demonstrate what was wanted, but they had such fine musical instincts and such an appreciation of voice that they produced beautiful results. Some of these individuals were excellent pianists and could illustrate dynamics and melodic line on the piano. Others had sufficient command of language to communicate their wishes through words and spoken inflection. Patience and empathy bring rich rewards.

INTONATION

A word should be said about intonation. For a thorough discussion, I refer you to the *Harvard Dictionary of Music* (Apel, 1965) and, in particular, the section on Intervals. Very briefly, a system of tuning known as *equal temperament* became common practice in Bach's time. In this, the scale was constructed of twelve equal intervals. *Just intonation* has been referred to as *nature's scale* because it contains three fundamental triads that are more pleasant in sound than either *Pythagorean* or *well-tempered* tuning. In modern music, with its modulation from key to key, *just intonation* would be quite useless. The following illustration (Figure XIV–2) shows why.

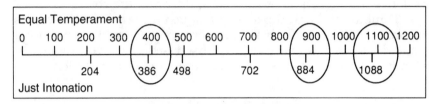

Figure XIV–2. In equal temperament, each half step is measured into 100 cents—a logarithmic measurement for scientific, exact method of measuring musical intervals. Notice that in "just intonation," the third, sixth and seventh of the scale are between 12 and 16 cents lower than for equal temperament.

In vocal music, whenever any part contains the 3rd, 6th, or 7th, they must be thought of as very high. This is especially true in choral music or the whole chorus will end up flat. Nature's scale will take over if you are not on your guard against it.

THE BEAUTY OF CHORAL SINGING

Many people derive satisfaction from participating in choral productions. The camaraderie, the sense of teamwork, the pleasure of mastering a difficult task, and the pride in bringing pleasure to others is hard to match. A number of voices singing together produces qualities and colors not possible with a solo voice. The beauty of tone from a well-balanced choir can mesmerize the ear as no other sounds are capable of doing. Perhaps, psychologically, it is symbolic of all humankind and, therefore, universal. Certainly, the great Bach oratorios reach to the very heights and depths of human feeling.

REFERENCES

Apel, W. (1965). *Harvard dictionary of music,* Cambridge, Ma: Harvard University Press.

XV

■

PHYSICAL FACTS

Singers will probably always rely heavily on sensation and imagery to guide them in vocal production, but a rudimentary understanding of the science of sound can enhance and facilitate the process. Such knowledge can help eliminate wasted effort and possible damage to the voice. In this chapter, I will lay out some aspects of physical science useful to voice teachers and their students.

Scientists and musicians use different terminology to describe the same physical phenomena. Table XV–1 gives a few definitions designed to bridge the gap.

THE MECHANICS OF SOUND

Sound is mechanical, radiant energy transmitted by the molecules in a medium such as air, water or wood plus a receiver for the sound to be heard. (There's the old question of whether a tree falling in a forest makes a sound if there is no one there to hear it.) At sea level and zero degrees centigrade, sound travels in air at the rate of 1088 feet per second in all directions, like light from a candle or a light bulb. Sound has no inherent ability to project in a single direction.

When the concept of "placing a tone" is mentioned, remember that 1088 ft. is more than 3½ times the length of a football field!

Table XV–1. Terminology Used by Scientists and Musicians

Physical (Scientific Term)	Perceptual (Musical Term)
Sound	**Sound**
Audible phenomena called *sound* have various discernible qualities which, when *measured*, are physical.	Audible phenomena with discernible qualities which, *when analyzed by the ear,* are perceptual.
Frequency	**Pitch**
Molecular energy—condensations and rarifactions.	Changes in frequency not always perceived as changes in pitch.
Intensity	**Loudness**
How far molecules move with what energy.	Indicated by terms of soft (quiet) and strong or big (loud).
Wave form	**Quality**
Composite of other attributes.	Timbre, described with words such as warm, hard, clear, or mellow.
Time	**Time**
Phase.	Duration.

FREQUENCY AND PITCH

When a scientist talks about frequency and a musician speaks about pitch, they are on the same subject. Frequency is expressed in hertz (Hz), a unit equal to one cycle per second. *Condensations* means that the molecules are closer together, *rarifactions* that they are further apart. *Pitch* is the lowness or highness of a note as perceived by the ear. Any sound wave that is not regular is called a *noise.*

The lowest tone discernible to the human ear is about 16 Hz, the highest about 20,000 Hz. The low A on the piano is 27.2 Hz; the highest note, C, is about 4,186 Hz. These figures are based on a standard of A = 440 Hz, the A above middle C.

The approximate pitch level for speech, averaging all males, is about C (130.8 Hz), one octave below middle C. For females it is one octave higher, at middle C. This refers to the "natural level" of a healthy voice rather than the "habitual level," which may be lower.

Frequency varies with changes of length, thickness, tension, and air pressure of or on the vibrating body. This is why such a wide range of pitches can be created by the vocal folds. On a violin, thinner strings produce higher sounds. If a string is tightened, its frequency increases. Thicker, looser strings produce lower tones.

The decibel level for two frequencies produced by the same energy force will be greater for the higher frequency. For example, let's suppose that two mezzos are singing two notes. One is singing middle C and the other is singing the G above it. Let's also assume that each is using the same amount of breath pressure. The G would measure more decibels (be louder) because it is higher. This explains why you might see a brass band with six sousaphones and just one piccolo.

Measured at the same distance on an intensity meter, the song of a canary shows the same intensity as the roar of a gorilla. Why do singers try to sing high tones loudly? If the notes are well produced, high tones need no amplification. (Reflect how nature has given small animals higher calls to allow them to give a cry of alarm as protection against larger animals with low growls.)

An increase in air pressure raises frequency in tones produced by a wind instrument. This law tells us that we should allow the vocal folds to adjust freely to the thought of pitch in order to avoid undue force for higher frequencies. Practicing scales from the bottom up without allowing the tone to become lighter and adjust for pitch is one of the most common practices in voice training. I have discussed this problem in further detail in Chapter III on Beginning Exercises.

BERNOULLI EFFECT

When you think of a pitch, your vocal folds begin to move together in the proper adjustment for that pitch. A flow of air finally draws them together. A physical law known as the *Bernoulli effect* states that moving air has less pressure than stationary air. Think of the tremendous suction created by a tornado or experiment by blowing between two pieces of paper held vertically in front of your lips. The papers represent the two vocal folds. I recommend selected writings by J. Van den Berg (1957) and William Vennard (1967) for more information on the Bernoulli effect. You may also wish to refer to Chapter IV for practical applications.

INTENSITY AND LOUDNESS

Intensity is the amount of energy or power per second per square centimeter of a sound wave. It diminishes rapidly with distance in space just like the circular ripples createrd by dropping a stone in still water. The intensity of a sound wave varies inversely as the square of the distance from the sound.

Scientists measue intensity in decibles (dB). One decibel equals the smallest change in loudness perceptible to the average listener. At zero decibels, no sound is heard. An ordinary conversation with speakers standing three feet apart is at about 65 dB. The loudest sound, the "threshold of pain," is about 120 dB. Musicians use the term intensity to convey a variety of meanings. For example, the word may be used to describe emotional impact as well as loudness, although loudness is indicated by terms of soft (quiet) and strong or big (loud).

When two equal tone sources are added together, the intensity (loudness) level is only increased by three decibels. For example, if two choirs of 40 voices were combined and each created an intensity of 60 dB, the combined choirs would produce only 63 dB. Add another choir of 80 voices to that 80 and you would have a potential of 66 dB of intensity. Doubling any quantity only adds three decibels.

If a soloist were singing with a choir but at higher pitches, the soloist would be heard because of the pitch differences. If the soloist were at the same pitch, but had developed a stronger "ring" in his voice, he would still be heard. The added resonance of the "ring" would increase the intensity beyond the intensity of any voice in the choir. Most soloists have this capacity.

VENTURI EFFECT

Another law of physics known as the *Venturi effect* states that the amount of pressure exerted by a substance flowing through an opening will vary according to the inverse square of that opening. The substance, in our case air, flowing through an opening, the glottis, will provide a greater subglottic pressure automatically if the opening is smaller (or firmer). For singers, this implies that the condition of the glottal opening is of greater importance than attempting to manipulate pressure from the lungs. If the glottis has gained the right kind of tonus in the vocal folds through training, not as much air will escape, the subglottal pressure will be greater and intensity will increase. I caution against any effort to make the glottis firmer. With proper exercise, the tonus or firmness of the vocal folds develops naturally over time .

Ordinarily intensity will vary according to the force with which air molecules are set in motion and will be perceived as degrees of loudness. Physiological control of intensity is conditioned upon the tension and firmness in the vocal folds and subglottal air pressure from the lungs.

WAVE FORM—QUALITY

The study of wave forms is very complex, especially when you get into the physical qualities that distinguish one vowel from another or those characteristics which produce the "ring" in resonance. In learning to sing, you should simply know that there are physical laws that determine how you produce tones, create firm sound, and form vowels at different frequencies and intensities. Let these laws work for you—don't fight them. Chapters VIII, IX, and X describe how to make use of these laws.

If the mass of a resonator is increased, the amount of resonance will increase. Resonance makes various sounds amplify differently. When sound is rebounded, there are reinforcements and cancellations of the various frequencies. Frequencies can be raised or lowered by altering the shapes through which they pass. This produces the changes in overtones in a voice called formants by which we distinguish various vowels even though the source of sound at the glottis is relatively constant.

As you watch actors on TV, notice how little you can see of all that is taking place as they form words. The tongue, jaw and muscles of the pharynx are performing a dance which makes vowels and consonants possible. Because we have been altering these spaces all our lives as we chew and swallow, we do not realize what is gong on.

Except for a pure sine wave, pitches consist of a fundamental frequency and overtones. The tone from a tuning fork produces a sine wave (pure tone). In contrast, if you strike the low C on the piano, while holding down the loud pedal, you can hear the overtones of C, an octave higher, the G above that, then the next C and the E a third above it. These are called overtones and are caused by divisions of the lowest string vibrating in segments. They do not stop at the E but are difficult to hear and isolate higher than that. An instrument called the spectrograph shows the higher overtones clearly. A simple test of this phenomenon is to place your finger lightly on the middle point between the two ends of a piano string. As you strike the key, you will hear a pitch one octave higher than the pitch of the free vibrating string.

RESONANCE

Webster (1981) defines resonance as (1) a vibration in a mechanical or electrical system caused by a relatively small periodic stimulus of the same or nearly the same period as the natural vibration of the system; (2) the intensification and enriching of a musical tone by supplementary vibration.

A tuning fork vibrating in the air is only lightly audible. If the lower end is set on a piece of wood, however, the entire body of wood is set into sympathetic vibration. As the air molecules surrounding the wood are disturbed, we perceive that the fork is making a much louder sound; yet, there is no more energy producing it. The energy all comes from the stroke that set the tuning fork in motion.

TIME

While a physicist cares not at all about how long you can hold a note, a musician concerns him- or herself with time signature, time value, and tempo.

BEAT PHENOMENON

You may notice what is known as a beat phenomenon when two vibrating sources differ only slightly in frequency. Anyone who has sung in a choir for a period of time has probably been aware of this but didn't know it had a name. It's the effect that you hear when someone next to you is just slightly sharp or flat from the frequency you are singing. As illustrated in Bartholomew's *Acoustics of Music* (1947), striking one tuning fork of 435 and another of 440 would produce beats at the rate of five per second as a result of alternately strengthening and weakening the resulting tone. Voices singing in unison must think their pitches very accurately to avoid an undesirable effect.

UNDERSTANDING PHYSICS OF SOUND CAN BE HELPFUL

If a voice doesn't seem to behave the way you think it should, a review of the physics of sound may help to focus on the problem. It is one of the aspects of sound making that many do not take into consideration.

REFERENCES

Bartholomew, W.T. (1947). *Acoustics of Music*, New York: Prentice-Hall.

Mirriam-Webster. (1981). *Eighth new collegiate dictionary.* Springfield, Ma: Mirriam-Webster.

Van den Berg, J., Zantema, J.T., & Doornenbal, P. (1957). *On the air resistance of the Bernoulli effect of the human larynx,* Journal of Acoustical Society of America, 29.

Vennard, W. (1967). *Singing, the mechanism and the technic,* New York: Carl Fischer, (pp. 166, 224, 240, 776, 901).

XVI

∎

LARYNGEAL ANATOMY
AND PHYSIOLOGY

Many will contend that the less you know about how your voice works, the better. I suggest that the more you understand the anatomy and physiology of voice production, the better equipped you will be to sing or to teach singing.

The descriptions in this chapter apply equally to male and female voices. They apply to all postpubescent voices, with the possible exception of those advanced in years. Because our concern is with building voices and maintaining good voice health during the active singing years, the special problems of elderly voices will not be discussed.

To understand many of the ideas presented in this book, you must bear in mind that humans are members of the animal kingdom. If you study the larynx from its evolutionary beginning, you learn that the lung fish, which spends part of its life on land, has a valvular mechanism which can open or close, depending on whether the fish is on land or in the water. The vocal folds in your throat are an outgrowth of the valvular mechanism of lower animal forms, such as the lung fish.

For its size, the larynx has been described as the most complex and versatile mechanical device in the body. What further complicates matters for a teacher is that "no one has been born or ever will be born who is exactly like anyone else, dead or alive" (*Anthropology Today*, 1971).

NINE FUNCTIONS OF THE VOCAL FOLDS

According to Jackson and Jackson (1937) the vocal folds have basically nine different functions. Briefly, they are as follows:

1. **Respiratory**: this serves in regulating interchange of carbon dioxide in the blood.
2. **Valvular**: a control which affects positive and negative pressure in the lungs; these in turn have an effect on pulmonary circulation.
3. **Fixative**: it stabilizes the thorax for efficient arm movement.
4. **Protective**: serves to prevent anything other than air from entering the air passages.
5. **Deglutitory**: it shuts off the airway so that no food or liquid can enter the lungs when you swallow.
6. **Tussive**: this is the cough that repels foreign bodies and keeps them from entering the larynx (e.g., dust, food particles).
7. **Expectorative**: its action clears the passage of secretions and inflammatory products from below the glottis level. (In other words, it clears your throat.)
8. **Emotional**: this function creates reflexive sounds such as crying, laughing, moaning, and so on. These sounds are considered phonatory, a continuous and even vibrating of the vocal folds, unlike a cough.
9. **Phonatory**: this is the voluntary use of sound as a means of communication.

These reflexive functions are as natural as those of your eyes, which focus automatically on objects far and near and adjust to different intensities of light. Some of the actions are quite vigorous, numbers 3 through 7, for example. Regarding number 6, the tussive function, in regions of the throat where airway compression occurs, gas velocities can range up to half or even three quarters of the speed of sound—between 300 and 400 miles per hour! Regarding number 3, the fixative function, in heavy arm work, your larynx will close. This closure stabilizes the breath pressure in your lungs and explains why people grunt when moving heavy objects. Obviously, this type of action does not go along with the free, open throat needed for singing.

What happens in the vocal folds to give such a wide range of frequencies and dynamics with so short and small a set of muscles? Excellent and complete descriptions of laryngeal muscle functions are given in books by Bunch (1982), Fink and Demarest (1978), Hirano et al. (1988), Sundberg (1987), Vennard (1967), Zemlin (1968), and others. What follows is a summary of findings I have found particularly relevant as a voice teacher.

LARYNGEAL FRAMEWORK

The principle framework of the larynx (see Figure XVI-1) consists of the following:

1. **The cricoid cartilage** is the lowest element in the larynx. Shaped like a signet ring with the broad portion posterior (at the back), it constitutes the top ring of the trachea.
2. **The two arytenoid cartilages** rest on the superior (upper) posterior (back) surface of the cricoid cartilage and are attached to it by ligaments and muscles.
3. **The thyroid cartilage**, which is open posteriorly, has two inferior (lower) horns and two superior horns. The inferior horns are attached to the external (outer) surfaces of the cricoid cartilage on either side by ligaments and muscles. The superior horns extend upward to attach to the hyoid bone by means of the lateral (side) thyroid ligaments. The anterior (front) angle of this cartilage is identifiable as the Adam's Apple. There is also a rim of thyrohyoid muscles.
4. **The hyoid bone**, at the top of the larynx, is shaped like a horseshoe with the opening posterior. Free from direct attachment to any other part of the body framework, this bone can move in any direction.

I only mention the presence of an epiglottis as well as two connuculate and two cuneiform cartilages (cartilages of Santorini and Wrisberg), because they seem to have no direct connection to laryngeal adjustments.

The cartilages of the larynx are suspended from the hyoid bone in a relationship that permits elastic motion at each point of articulation. The laryngeal ligaments have been compared to coiled

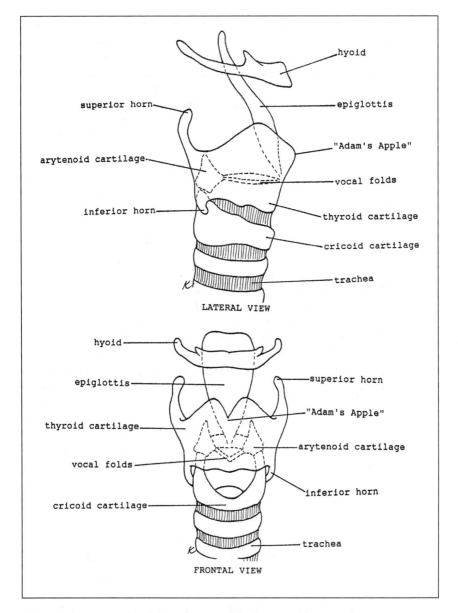

Figure XVI–1. Lateral and frontal views of the laryngeal framework.

springs that can rest, be compressed, or stretched, permitting a number of antagonistic actions.

INTRINSIC LARYNGEAL MUSCLES

These muscles are attached only to the laryngeal framework (see Figure XVI–2a, b, c, and d).

1. **Thyroarytenoid** muscles (Figure XVI–2a) are the two vocal folds, consisting of external and internal divisions and vocal ligament. They extend posteriorly from the inner surface of the thyroid notch (Adam's Apple) to their attachments to each of the two arytenoid cartilages at what is known as the vocal process and the body of the arytenoid. These folds are covered by a thin mucous lining called the epithelium, which is free to move over the underlying muscles much as the skin on the back of your hand can slide over the tissues beneath. The epithelium is part of the mucous lining which covers the inner surfaces of the entire laryngeal tract from the nose down through the mouth, pharynx, and larynx to the trachea.

    When the folds contract, they shorten and thicken; when relaxed, they can be stretched. They separate the most in the mid-dle of the glottis for inspiration of air and may be approximated (drawn together) for other functions, such as phonation.

2. **The posterior cricoarytenoids** are a pair of muscles that abduct (separate) the vocal folds. These muscles rise from the posterior surface of the cricoid cartilage and insert into the posterior area of the muscular processes of the arytenoids. Their action opens the glottis for the intake of air. In forced inspirations the glottis may be opened almost twice the average opening of 8 mm in males.

3. **The lateral cricoarytenoids** are a pair of muscles that adduct (draw together) the vocal folds and close the glottis by drawing the muscular processes of the arytenoids toward a midline. They rise from the upper borders of the cricoid cartilage on either side and insert into the anterior area of the muscular processes of the arytenoids. Their contraction rotates the arytenoids forward. In extreme action, they carry the entire arytenoids a bit forward, producing the posterior opening characteristic of the whisper.

4. **The interarytenoids**, considered as a single muscle, close the posterior opening between the arytenoids. This muscle runs from the posterior, lateral surface of one arytenoid to the other. A transverse portion draws the median margins

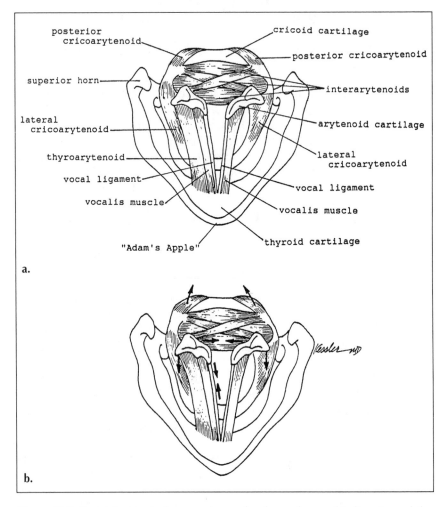

Figure XVI–2. (a) Instrinsic laryngeal muscles from above; (b) direction of the muscle action; *(continued)*

of the arytenoids together while an oblique portion acts on the topmost angle, called the apex.

5. **The cricothyroid** muscles (Figure XVI–2c) have two parts, the *pars recta* and the *pars obliqua.* The pars recta serves to approximate (draw together) the thyroid and cricoid cartilages anteriorly, with the inferior horns of the thyroid cartilage acting as a fulcrum. This action elongates, and tenses

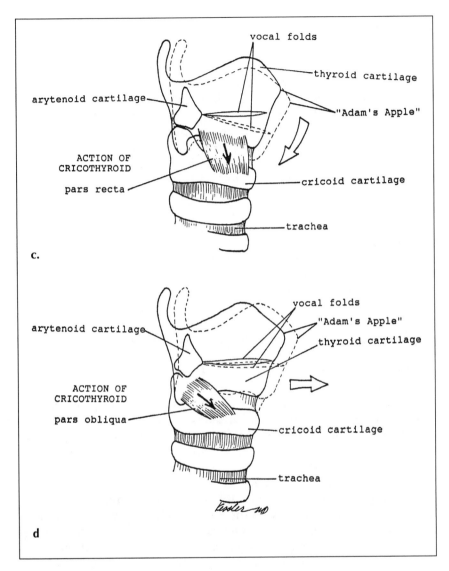

Figure XVI–2. *(continued)*
(c & d) cricothyroid muscles and the effect of their actions on the vocal folds.

the vocal folds, which are suspended between the thyroid
cartilage and the arytenoids. The pars obliqua puts a
further stretch on the vocal folds by pulling the inferior
horns of the thyroid cartilage forward in a gliding motion

from their ligamentous attachments to the cricoid cartilage. I call these the singer's muscles.

Since the arytenoids sit on the cricoid, they rock along with it. In addition, their attachments to the cricoid cartilage allows them to slide laterally as well as tilt forward and back.

Freedom of motion is the key to free phonation. The actions of the intrinsic muscles of the larynx are directly associated with the vocal folds. They contribute to vocal production by closing the glottis for phonation and opening it for the intake of air. Pitch variations are made by shortening and thickening, or lengthening and thinning the vocal folds. Lower notes are produced by shortening and thickening the vocal folds, which involves somewhat complex vibrations of the entire length, depth, and width of the vocal folds.

An examination of the folds shows that they are deeper than they are wide. In normal phonation, when looking through a laryngeal mirror, you see only the superior surface of the folds, partly obscured by the ventricular bands which lie superior to the true folds. If you look at a laminogram of the folds from the front you can see that they extend inferiorly to a greater degree than they do laterally.

As the vocal folds adjust to create lower tones, a broader surface of the epithelium meets at midline. Getting back to one of the physical concepts presented in the preceding chapter, remember that an increase in mass and a decrease in tension lowers the frequency of a sound. The vocal folds can create considerable effects, therefore, with great economy. By comparison, the violin employs four strings of varying thickness in addition to adjustments for tension for its range of frequencies.

For higher frequencies, greater tension is exerted on the folds from front to back. At the same time, the folds become thinner vertically, leaving only the thinned upper edges to vibrate. This is achieved principally by the action of the cricothyroid muscles in coordination with a decreased action of the thyroarytenoids.

When the fibers of a muscle are activated, they shorten; when they relax, they can be stretched by other muscles. If you tighten your biceps, they thicken and shorten. If you relax them, they become loose and are subject to lengthening from the pull of other muscles.

A possible added tensor of the vocal folds is the downward and backward force exerted on the arytenoids by the contraction of the posterior cricoarytenoids. Just how much they contribute has been difficult to measure.

For frequency adjustments, the intrinsic muscles function from the level of the thyroid cartilage downward. To permit this, extrinsic muscles, which can exert an upward pull, must be as free as possible from unnecessary activity during phonation. Because the vocal folds are suspended between three different cartilages, extrinsic muscle action can impede free movement of the intrinsic muscles and impede their adjustments for phonation.

Bear in mind that the whole laryngeal unit from the hyoid bone down through the cricoid cartilage is suspended within the neck. This allows for elastic movements up and down, side to side and, to a lesser degree, front to back. The larynx, being linked to the trachea below is sensitive to action in the whole upper body. Above, the larynx opens into the pharynx, mouth, and all other parts of the head. Specifically, because the whole laryngeal area is so closely associated with the human voice, much emphasis is placed on finding as much freedom as possible in all its parts.

EXTRINSIC LARYNGEAL MUSCLES

Much less is known about the affect of the extrinsic muscles (see Figure XVI–3) on phonation. They can exert numerous pulls on the hyoid bone and cartilages of the larynx, working together under the best conditions and at cross purposes under others.

Following Zemlin's (1968) classification, I list ten extrinsic muscles, one on each side of the neck, for a total of twenty:

1. The **sternohyoid** muscles insert into the manubrium sterni and clavicles and extend upward to the lower body of the hyoid bone. Their action lowers the hyoid bone and helps to stabilize the larynx in loud singing.
2. The **sternothyroid** muscles also insert into the manubrium sterni and extend to the thyroid cartilage. Recent research indicates that many of the fibers in these muscles originate in the consecutive tissue of the upper portion of the fibrous pericardium, a tissue surrounding the heart and having connections to the diaphragm. This could affect laryngeal position by drawing the larynx downward on inspiration because of the contraction of the diaphragm. These muscles work with the sternohyoid in stabilizing the larynx.
3. The **omohyoid** muscles insert into the upper border of the scapula (shoulder blade), which explains, in part, why stiff

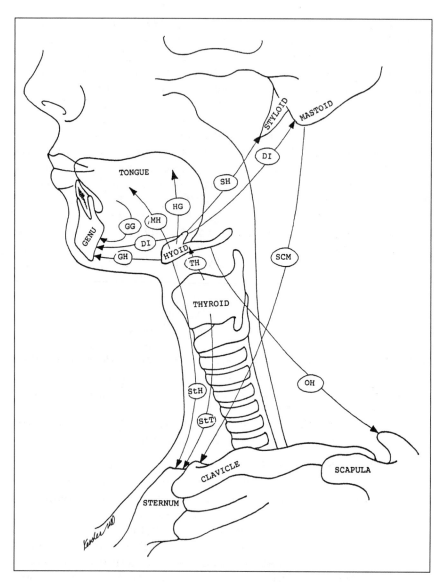

Figure XVI–3. Extrinsic laryngeal muscles and the direction of their action. GG, genioglossus; DI, diagastric; GH, geniohyoid; MH, mylohyoid; HG, hyoglossus; SH, stylohyoid; TH, thyrohyoid; StH, sternohyoid; StT, sternothyroid; OH, omohyoid; SCM, sternocleidomastoid.

shoulders affect freedom of movement in the larynx. The lower "belly" of each omohyoid muscle inserts into a tendon behind the sterno-cleidomastoid. From here, the upper belly extends upward and inserts into the lower border of the hyoid bone. These muscles lower and draw back the hyoid bone and the larynx.

4. The **thyrohyoid** muscles extend from the oblique line of the thyroid cartilage to the lower border and greater horn of the hyoid bone. Their action decreases the distance between the thyroid cartilage and the hyoid bone. The negative effect this has on the free adjustments of the vocal folds can be countered, in part, by the sensation of letting your larynx hang loosely.

5. The **digastric** muscles have an anterior and a posterior belly. The anterior belly extends from the inside of the mandible down and back to an intermediate tendon on the greater cornu (horn) of the hyoid bone. From here, the posterior belly goes back to the mastoid notch of the temporal bone. Their action can raise the hyoid bone or help to lower the jaw. Jaw tension tends to pull your larynx up.

6. The **stylohyoid** muscles extend from the styloid processes of the temporal bone down and forward to the hyoid bone, just above the omohyoid insertion. They draw the hyoid bone up and back.

7. The **geniohyoid** muscles extend from the back of the mandible to the anterior surface of the hyoid bone. They can elevate the hyoid bone, drawing it forward. To help the larynx rest in a lower position, check under your chin for looseness.

8. The **genioglossus** muscles also originate from the back of the mandible. Their lower fibers insert into the hyoid bone and their upper fibers insert along the whole under surface of the tongue to its tip. Their action can draw the hyoid bone forward and protrude the tongue. It can also affect tongue tension.

9. The **hyoglossus** muscles rise from the upper border of the hyoid bone and insert into the back and sides of the tongue. Tension may inhibit the free positioning of the larynx.

10. The **mylohyoid** muscles extend from the mylohyoid line of the mandible to the hyoid bone. They can raise the hyoid bone, tongue, and floor of the mouth if the mandible is fixed. A stiff jaw will definitely inhibit the free positioning of the larynx.

Research published by Aatto Sonninen (1956) in the 1950s is still helpful. More recently, however, research by Estill, Baer, Honda, and others (1983) documents the effect of some of the supralaryngeal muscles on six voice qualities, including "belt" and "opera." Illustrations of the extrinsic muscles indicate the complexity of the laryngeal system. Note that more muscles act to raise than to lower the larynx. Swallowing lifts and closes the larynx to prevent food from entering the trachea and to guide food down the esophagus.

Intermingled with the extrinsic muscles are the muscles of the tongue, palate, muscles of chewing, and muscles of the face. For example, when a person changes expression on his face, muscles in his pharynx respond reflexively.

If the intrinsic muscles of the larynx are to be free for automatic adjustment to the thought of a pitch, then the extrinsic muscles must be in a condition of what I term *release*. Interfering actions may be acquired through misconceptions, unnatural tasks, or an environment that inhibited normal development. Rest assured that every healthy individual has all the natural endowments with which he or she was born. If you add to this the fact that each individual's muscles, cartilages, ligaments, and bones are different and that each person has a different number of muscle fibers, it becomes quite obvious why no two people can produce the same sound and why physical sensations of what is happening when the voice is used will vary from individual to individual.

Knowing about the anatomy and physiology of the larynx should help you to free your voice and allow it to grow in a natural manner. Thinking the desired pitch and freeing the muscles to perform their functions require trust. You must learn to trust that what you want to have happen will happen if you let it. Developing this kind of trust may be the hardest part of learning to sing.

REFERENCES

Anthropology Today. (1971). Ed. Roe, R. L., Del Mar, Ca: Communications Research Machines, Inc.

Bunch, M. (1982). *Dynamics of the singing voice*, New York: Springer-Verlag.

Estill, J., Baer, T. Honda, H., Kiyoshi, H. & Harris, K. S. (1983). An EMG study of supralaryngeal activity in six voice qualities. *Transcripts of the 12th Symposium*, Care of the professional voice, Part I, New York: The Voice Foundation.

Fink, B. R., & Demarest, R. J. (1978). *Laryngeal biomechanics*, Cambridge, Ma: Harvard University Press.

Hirano, M., Kiyokawa K., & Kurita, S. (1988). *Laryngeal muscles and glottic shaping*, Vocal Fold Physiology, (Vol. 2), New York: Raven Press.

Jackson, C., & Jackson, C. L., Jr. (1937). *The larynx and its diseases*, Philadelphia, Pa: Saunders.

Sonninen, A. A. (1956). The role of the external laryngeal muscles in length of adjustment of the vocal cords in singing. Helsinki: *Acta Oto-Laryngologia.*

Sundberg. J. (1987). *The science of the singing voice*, Dekalb, Il: Northern Illinois University Press.

Vennard, W. (1967). *Singing, the mechanism and the technic*, New York: Carl Fischer.

Zemlin, W. (1968). *Speech and hearing science*, Englewood Cliffs, NJ: Prentice-Hall.

XVII

■

NEUROLOGY AND
THE BRAIN

Imagine arriving in New York City a complete stranger and using a subway map to find your way around. That map, complex in its own right, would be only a fraction (one thousandth of one percent) as complex as a map of the human nervous system. Even if you could follow a map of the nervous system, research begun little more than twenty years ago is advancing so quickly, the map might be deemed obsolete the moment it was handed to you.

Though I am no authority on the human nervous system, I have found bits of information from neurological science that deepened my understanding of how we make sound and the ways we control the sounds we make. In this chapter on neurology and the brain, I will attempt to share the information I have gathered with you.

THE COMMAND CENTER

Singing requires thinking. You have to think pitches (frequencies), time values (duration, phase), tempo (speed), dynamics (intensity, degrees of loudness), mood (wave form, emotional context)—in fact, everything you do. Your brain controls your thinking and remembering and gives commands to your muscles. Your voice responds to mental concepts which are accumulations of what you have heard, read, felt, seen, imagined, or experienced. As

Judson and Weaver (1965) explain in their text *Voice Science*, these concepts are holistic, "it is the high level of neurological control that has permitted man to speak" (p. 230).

Your brain contains between ten billion and one hundred billion cells, more cells than there are stars in our galaxy. The number of neuronal connections in the brain is perhaps ten to the fifteenth power (10^{15}). Brain cell multiplication during the nine months before birth are at the rate of about 250,000 new neurons per minute (Restak, 1984, p. 42). In his book, *Mega Brain*, Michael Hutchinson (1986) writes, "all evidence indicates that whether we are twenty, forty or eighty, our brains have the capability of growing and we have the ability to become more intelligent" (p. 55). In a similar vein, Douglas Starr (1984) has written, "It's what you do—not when you do it . . . . Benjamin Franklin was a newspaper columnist at 16 and a framer of the United States Constitution at 81. William Pitt became prime minister of Great Britain at 24 and George Bernard Shaw was 94 when one of his plays was first produced. Age has little to do with ability."

A 1986 article on memory in *Newsweek* (September 29, p. 48) stated that, "before there is knowledge, there must be memory. Some sections of the mind's archives store facts (names, images, events) while others store procedures (how to do things). Samuel Johnson once said that the true art of memory is the art of attention." Pay attention to what your body is doing when your voice is functioning the way you want it to. Much benefit is gained by observing how your body operates and remembering what your sensations were. You learned to speak by remembering the significance of "mama" and translating that sound from the unconscious to the conscious area of the brain.

THE NERVOUS SYSTEM

The nervous system carries messages to the brain and from the brain back through your body to the proper organs and muscles for action. Some responses are chemical, such as the release of adrenaline into the bloodstream. Others are carried by nerve fibers to muscles which contract in response to stimuli.

To state it in the simplest possible terms, you have a voluntary and an involuntary nervous system. Voluntary impulses are processed by the thinking part of the brain, the top part, the cortex, developed in the latest phase of our evolution as human beings. The involuntary nervous system, sometimes called the autonomic nervous system, serves many functions without our direct attention.

The oldest, most primitive part of the nervous system is the spinal cord. When you touch something hot, you immediately pull your finger away without any impulse going to your brain. It all takes place in a matter of milliseconds.

At the base of the brain and directly connected to the spinal cord is the *medulla oblongata*, which serves to carry out the processes of such brain functions as swallowing, breathing, control of blood pressure, talking, singing, and, in part, heart rate. An involuntary laugh or cry is triggered at this point. Only a short distance above the medulla is the *hypothalamus*, which integrates behaviors related to emotional states (Figure XVII-1). The fact that the larynx has a direct connection to the medulla has many interesting implications which will be considered in Chapter XIX on Enigmas.

A neuron is commonly regarded as the functional unit of the central nervous system. It has extensions classified as *axons* and *dendrites*, the axons conducting impulses away from the cell body and the dendrites conducting impulses toward it (Figure XVII-2).[1] It may be useful to think of a neuron as a telephone operator who receives and transmits messages. A stimulus, such as seeing a note on a sheet of music sends that information by way of an *afferent nerve fiber* to the neuron which receives it through its incoming connection called a dendrite. If the note was to be played on a piano, the neuron would send a message through its outgoing connection, an axon, along *efferent nerve fibers* to the muscle or muscles needed to position and activate a response in the correct finger to play that note. The neuron "operator" has many outlets available at its switchboard. It will only act, however, if it has sufficient stimulus to do something. For example, the note could have been seen but the person had no desire to play it, remember it, or give it significance in any way—in which case nothing would happen.

When you have seen and played a series of notes frequently, it is no longer necessary to work out the fingering because the neuron has made the connection so many times that it has

---

[1] I am indebted to Jacques Acar, MD, for the original concepts of Figures XVII-1 and XVII-3.

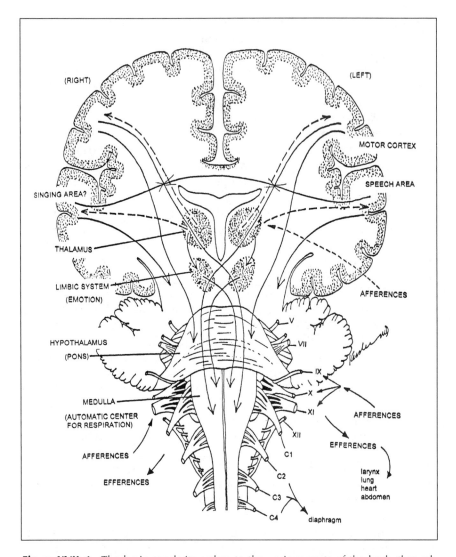

Figure XVII–1. The brain sends its orders to the various parts of the body through the *efferent nervous system.*

relegated the task to an assistant as a routine action no longer needing special attention. This lower level of response is known as a *reflex arc* or a *conditioned reflex*. This is the level of activity that you should strive to bring about in your study of singing.

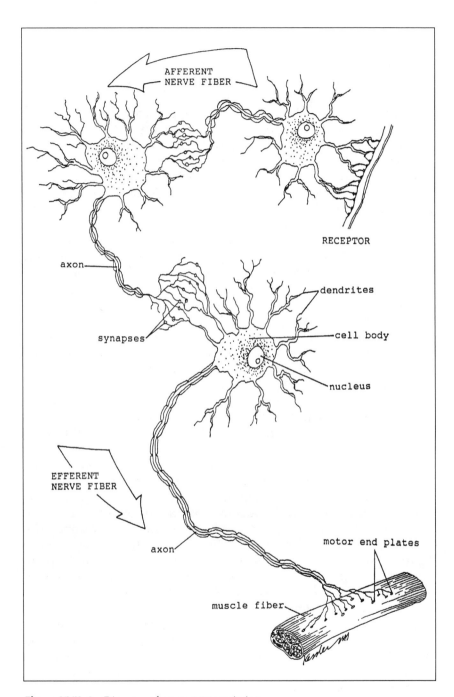

Figure XVII–2. Diagram of neuron transmission.

One nerve fiber may divide to supply as many as 150 muscle fibers in some muscles or 400 fibers in others. In addition, the nerve to a muscle may contain fibers from several sections of the spinal cord. Some believe that the ratio of axons to muscle fibers in the thyroarytenoid is as low as 1 : 1.

To remain in healthy condition, the nerves need to be called upon regularly. If they are not used on a routine basis, nerves can atrophy. It's the old story, if you don't use it, you lose it. On the other hand, when you are concentrating and striving to do your utmost, a maximum number of nerve endings are stimulated and your greatest efficiency, known as a *point of saturation* is reached. Here, we meet our old friend, our sixth sense, proprioception. Proprioceptive nerve fibers conduct afferent sensations from muscles, tendons, ligaments, and joints to the brain. Through a connection with the inner ear, they also affect your sense of balance. These sensations are essential to your awareness of the position, condition, and movement of the many mechanisms within your body. As you will see, they are of great importance to singers.

Conscious impulses originate in the top of the brain. Many actions can take place at a subconscious level by means of the reflex arc. The neural connection for both responses is known as a *synapse*. There is a space between the axon and the efferent nerve fiber across which neurological impulses jump much the same as a spark jumps from the end of one wire to another under the right conditions. That "jump" depends on your having sufficient stimulus to want to do something.

The lungs, as well as being controlled by the autonomic nervous system, have a direct connection from the cortex motor neurons to the spinal cord neurons in the thoracic region of the body. Control over the breathing mechanism can therefore be developed by observing what happens in normal breathing. The British physiologist Charles Phillips has postulated that these "brain-to-spinal-cord connections are probably related not to respiration but to the use of respiratory muscles in such skilled activities as speech and song" (in Evarts, 1979, p. 172).

Humans can promote conscious actions for speech and song because of our high level of brain development, a skill not available to lower animals. By establishing specific motions through a routine of repeated practice terms, these actions can eventually be relegated to the reflex centers, thus leaving the mind free to concentrate on other objectives.

Think how remarkable it is that a child, left on his own, will learn to walk. His body teaches him how to do it. It is the same in learning to ride a bicycle, walk a tightrope, or juggle several objects. You sensitize kinesthetic responses to become reflexes through repeated efforts to accomplish a particular act.

Through practice, you can develop a *pre-phonatory inspiration* equal to the task that the breath has to carry out. In the same way, by thinking very carefully what pitch you want to sing, a *pre-phonatory set of the laryngeal muscles* occurs—the muscles adjust to your thought of a pitch (Wyke, 1979, p. 46). Both of these require great concentration. Concentration is also required for you to think and feel a condition of an open, free, relaxed throat that is ready to speak or sing.

Most of the proprioceptive impulses occur at a subconscious level and are called *kinesthetic senses*. To ensure proper muscle tone and coordination for singing, however, the cerebellar cortex must have proprioceptive information.

There are receptor systems throughout the respiratory tract and larynx, including nerve endings in the laryngeal tissue. These systems are also present in the tissue below the larynx and respond to changes in breath pressure. The afferent nerves send impulses to the brain, giving information on how well you are adjusting your muscles for the actions you are thinking. The brain can quickly send messages back for any adjustments that might be needed.

An illustration of how the nerves carry this information to the brain can be seen in Figure XVII–1. Notice in this depiction how the stimuli from one side of the body affects the opposite side of the brain. It has been found that speech depends primarily on the left side of the brain while music depends on the right side. The emotions also seem to be involved with the right brain. This close relationship between music and the emotions is an interesting area for speculation. A crossover combining both hemispheres is needed for singing, since both words and music are employed. Fortunately, within the brain, messages can be carried back and forth from one side to the other.

It has already been mentioned that below the hypothalamus are those parts of the brain and spinal cord which control the reflexes and the automatic body functions. There are sections just above the primitive part of the brain which control such higher functions as sensation, language, planning, and thought. Through *biofeedback*, people seek to control reactions mediated by the hypothalamus. Investigations are constantly enlarging our knowledge of how this is done.

As already stated, the signaling system from the neuron is both electrical and chemical. Another most important means by which mind and body communicate is through the *endocrine system*. The endocrine system needs the nervous system for many of its functions. *Hormones* are a substance that move processes of the body. They organize responses to changing environments both inside and outside the body. The level of hormones circulated by the endocrine system is controlled by a negative feedback that keeps the various functions in balance— neither too little nor too much.

THE NERVES INVOLVED WITH SINGING

Singing involves the whole body. Figure XVII–3 shows how the fibers for several different functions share the same nerve branch. For clarity of identification, the various nerves have been separated so that they appear as individual branches rather than being intertwined in a single trunk as they appear in real life.

One of the nerves, number X, the *Vagus*, is also referred to as the *laryngeal nerve*. This nerve rises by several roots from the medulla oblongata. The *superior branch* serves the cricothyroid muscles. The *inferior portion* controls the posterior cricoary-tenoids, the lateral cricoarytenoids, the thyroarytenoids and the interarytenoids. You can see that it has not only these superior and inferior branches, but also branches that go to the stomach and heart. In addition, there are links between the nucleus of the Xth and the spinal nerve, XI, and, indirectly, the phrenic (dia-phragm) and all spinal nerves, including the clavicular.

The inferior branches of Nerve number X, the *recurrent laryngeal* nerve, run low into the chest area, the left branch lower than the right. It runs almost to the bottom of the sternum. Pressure from an enlarged heart or other abnormal conditions in this locale can affect this nerve and therefore the voice. Trauma to this nerve, which might happen inadvertently during surgery, for example, could also affect the voice.

The IXth or *glossopharyngeal nerve* has more than three links to the vagus nerve and roots in the medulla. Sensations from the mucous membrane of the pharynx, the pillars of the fauces, the posterior part of the tongue, as well as the stylo-

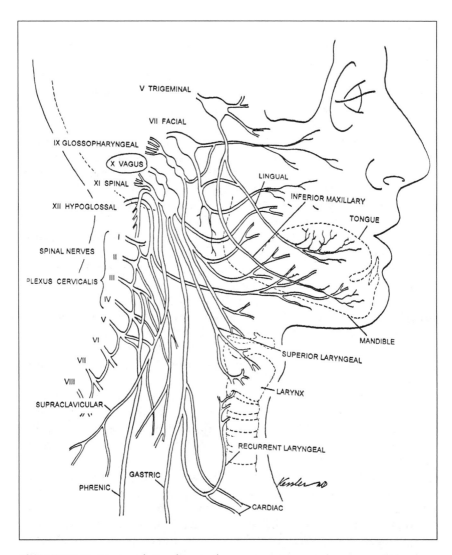

Figure XVII–3. Nerve relationships to the vagus nerve.

pharyngeus muscles are carried by this nerve. The value of the instruction to "have the sensation of the beginning of a yawn" takes on considerable meaning when you become aware of what might be taking place in this part of the vocal tract as you respond.

The VIIth nerve is called the *facial nerve*. It also arises from the medulla and serves the stylohoid, the posterior portion of the digastricus, the upper and lower muscles of the face, the lower lip, and the chin. The fact that some teachers want students to have the expression of a slight smile recognizes the connection between the muscles of the face and tone quality. Implications for the use of this knowledge are numerous. It has been said that we have two means of communicating feelings: facial expressions and the voice.

The Vth nerve arises from the pons, close to the medulla, and serves the mylohyoid, the anterior belly of the digastricus, the soft palate, the teeth, tongue, and the masseter or large chewing muscles closing the jaw. You may have experienced a change in your voice when you had a toothache or burned your tongue.

It is interesting to observe the effect of an immobilized jaw on the tongue. Place your hands on your jaw to become aware of any motion and, as if your hands were not holding your jaw, try to say something. It's as bad as trying to respond when your dentist has both hands in your mouth! A loose jaw induces a loose tongue.

The XIth nerve originates in the medulla and also the cervical part of the spinal cord. It innervates the trapezeus and the sternocleidomastoid muscles. Notice its strong link with the vagus nerve. You can see how important it is for the shoulders and neck muscles to be relaxed and free. (The trapezius covers the upper, back part of the neck and shoulder. The upper part of one side draws the head toward the same side and turns the face in the opposite direction. Both sides together draw the head directly backward. The sternocleidomastoid passes obliquely across the side of the neck. It draws the head toward the same side and points the chin upward to the opposite side.)

The XIIth nerve arises from the anterior of the medulla and serves the genioglossus, hyoglossus, geniohyoid, and other extrinsic muscles. (The hyoglossus runs from the sides of the hyoid bone to the sides of the tongue.) It is very important for tongue motions in articulation. If this nerve is paralyzed, the tongue cannot move. On the other hand, hyperfunction caused by the nerve can have an adverse effect on the mobility of the larynx because of the attachments of the base of the tongue to the hyoid bone.

Of the spinal nerves, the first four are more sensitive to disturbance in the larynx due to their connection with the hypoglossal nerve XII. Nerves V through VIII serve the lower part of the ribs and back. All the cervical nerves, however, are associated with respiration in one way or another and therefore affect the production of speech and song. Injury to any part of the spine can seriously inhibit freedom in breathing and thus seriously affect phonation.

In addition to all the above, you possess a *sympathetic nervous system* by which an injury to one part of the body can excite responses in another organ. For example, one day while walking down a corridor, I met a college professor who was an excellent public speaker. He was limping as he approached, so I asked him what had happened. In a very pained and strained voice, he replied, "I stepped on a nail!" Why did his voice have such a strained quality when the injury was in the bottom of his foot? It was his sympathetic nervous system at work.

You also have an *empathetic nervous system* which reacts to stimuli outside your body. I have described the experience of leaving a concert hall with an aching throat after hearing someone sing in a pushed or strained manner. The same empathetic response occurs when you have a conversation with someone who is angry. It is only with the greatest self-control that you can restrain from replying in a similar angry tone. In other words, your empathetic nervous system prompts you to respond in kind. A smile begets a smile—aggression induces aggression. Remember this when performing with others. Through empathy, it is possible to explore what others are experiencing. Developed to a high degree, it is one of the most valuable tools of a singing teacher.

MUSCLES AND THE NERVOUS SYSTEM

Muscles contain *slow-twitch* motor units with great resistance to fatigue, and *fast-twitch* units which generate large peak muscle tension but fatigue rapidly. Slow-twitch units are the first to be called upon, with fast-twitch units coming in last but tiring quickly. These facts give pause for thought as to how you can get the fullest benefits in the procedures for voice exercise. Singers are long distance athletes and need to conserve energy for the climaxes.

Muscle movements occur in response to the central nervous system. It is virtually impossible to contract a single muscle at will, the action more often being a part of a group response. Different actions may originate from within the same muscle. The greater the muscle action, the larger the number of muscle fibers that are stimulated within the bundle. Every muscle action is opposed by an antagonistic action (your lower arm is lifted by the biceps and extended by the triceps).

Human beings have a capacity for self-awareness that is not shared by the rest of the animal kingdom. Our reactions to our environment are complex because of our higher mental capacity, and we are impressionable at many different levels.

USING YOUR REFLEXES AND YOUR EXPERIENCES

The study of voice unavoidably brings one to consider experiences that predate your study. Depending on what those experiences were, you may bring a relatively simple set of vocal patterns to your study or complicated ones. These could be associated with speech or other sounds made in the past. Your old habits can make the process of learning to sing easy or complex. If something seems to be interfering with your learning, you should trace the source of the difficulty, not overlooking anything anywhere in the body.

I have often compared the kind of concentration needed for singing to the skill required in a game of darts. You must concentrate on the target, take careful aim, move your arm and snap your wrist with just the right amount of energy, and then let go! Through practice, the aim and control of energy in the release become more and more precise. In singing, as in darts, you must release the sound and hit the target.

A student performing in England was invited by a friend to try a game of darts. Having never played before, he asked what he was supposed to do. He was told that he must throw the dart and try to hit the center of the target. He looked at the bull's eye, picked up the dart, and let it fly. Right on! Again and again he made high scores, to everyone's surprise, not least his own. Several days later he thought he would perfect his game, since he did so well the first time. The harder he tried to make it perfect, the less well he did. He didn't trust his instincts, his body knowledge! All of us need to learn to keep out of our own way, to develop a trust in what our minds and bodies can do.

To summarize, perhaps the most valuable lesson you can learn from this chapter is that the laws of reflex action, which have long been known to operate at the level of the spinal cord motor neurons, also operate at the level of the motor cortex during volitional movements. "The actual events that underlie the achievement of the goal are built up from a variety of reflex processes" Wyke (1979, p. 42). As William James wrote some hundred years ago, "The marksman ends by thinking of the exact position of the goal, the singer only of the perfect sound" (in Evarts, 1979, p. 179). The hardest part is to trust the easiest way to do it.

REFERENCES

Evarts, E. V. (1979, September). *Brain mechanisms of movement*, Scientific American (p. 172).

Hutchinson, M. (1986). *Mega brain*, New York: Beech Tree Books (p. 55).

Judson, L. S. V., & Weaver, A. T. (1965). *Voice Science*, New York: Appleton-Century-Croft (p. 230).

Memory (1986, September 29). Article in *Newsweek*.

Restak, R. W. (1984). *The Brain*, New York: Bantam Books (p. 42).

Starr, D. A. (1984, June). *A window on the brain*, Readers Digest, (p. 100).

Wyke, B. (1979). Neurological aspects of phonatory control systems in the larynx; a review of current concepts. *Transcripts of the 8th Symposium, Part II, Care of the professional voice*, New York: The Voice Foundation (p. 42).

XVIII

■

HEARING

"Will they hear me if I sing like that? Is that all I have to do?"
I've heard those questions so many times! And I understand why students ask, especially about their high notes. This is
one of the particular reasons for including this chapter.

I am not attempting to present a complete thesis on hearing
by any means. Nor will I go into the anatomy and physiology. If
you want that approach, I suggest you read Zemlin's (1968)
Speech and Hearing Science. The points I have selected will be of
particular interest to teachers and singers seeking a broader
understanding of healthy voice use.

WHAT IS HEARING

Hearing is the special sense by which noises and tones are received
as stimuli. Sound is transmitted through the air by molecules.
When one molecule is stimulated, it passes that energy on to the
next molecule in a chain reaction. You could compare this
phenomenon to a row of dominoes, each passing along the little
push given to the first one—except that a molecule would return to
its original position. When the sound wave reaches the molecule
nearest your eardrum, the energy is transmitted into nerve impulses that are carried to your brain and recognized as sound.
Through experience, you attribute meaning to various sounds.

The unit for recording the relative intensity (loudness) of sound
has already been defined as a *decibel (db)*, the smallest change in

197

intensity (loudness) that can be recognized by your ear. A decibel change in intensity is a measure of the change in energy that it took to produce the sound. When someone yells at you, they have put more intensity (energy) into their voice than in soft speech and your ear hears it at a level of more decibels. In review, the "threshold" of hearing is designated as 0 db, the point where you can just hear a tone. The most you can hear safely is called the "threshold of pain," and is measured at approximately 120 db.

Frequency (pitch) is measured in hertz (Hz), or cycles per second of a vibrating element. The lowest sound that can be heard as a pitch is between 16 and 20 Hz. Anything lower is just a rumble. In the lowest tones of an organ you can even feel the vibrations. The highest tones that can be heard are between 16,000 and 20,000 Hz.

Figure XVIII–1 shows the average response of the normal ear to sounds of different frequencies. This chart is the result of

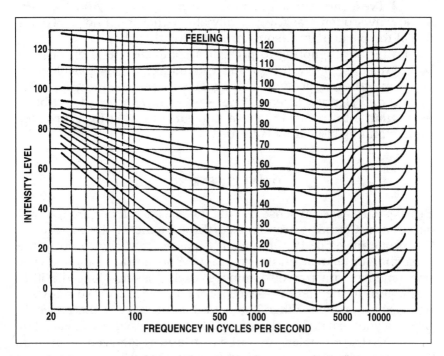

Figure XVIII–1. Loudness level curves. From *Musical Acoustics* (p. 33), by C. A. Culver, 1941, Philadelphia, Pa; The Blakiston Co.

extensive research by engineers of the Bell Laboratories at the New York World's Fair in the late 1930s (Culver, 1941). It shows clearly and simply how your ear responds to different frequencies (pitches) and intensities (loudness). If third space C on the piano were 512 Hz and played just loud enough so that you could hear it, the intensity (energy) to produce it would be about 5 db. The lowest C on the piano is 32 Hz. Looking at the chart, you can see that this would need an energy (intensity) of 60 db for you to hear it. It's hard to believe, but facts are facts. I have already used the analogy of how many sousaphones it would take in a brass band to balance just one piccolo.

Notice on the chart that your ear is most sensitive to sounds in the frequency range between 700 and 7000 Hz, the peak being at about 2500 Hz. This pitch of 2500 Hz is close to the E above high C, the third line above the staff. This explains why high sopranos do not need to sing their high notes loudly. Your larynx can produce high pitches with what feels like very light adjustments.

It may seem confusing to you that it takes more energy to produce an audible low note than an audible high note when we know that producing high notes requires greater compression. But, the action of the ear in response to sound and the mechanics of producing a sound are two distinct processes. Try to keep the two separate in your mind. Your ear responds to high frequencies much more sensitively than to low ones. Study the chart carefully.

To help put these hearing sensations into perspective, it is estimated that at a distance of three feet, ordinary conversation will be at a level of 65 db. Loud music in your home may be 80 db. The noise in a New York subway could be 95 db, while the sounds from a full symphony orchestra might range from 25 to 95 db (Bartholomew, 1942). The Walkman-type stereo, developed by Sony in 1979, can produce volume levels to 100 db. This corresponds to the noise level of a pneumatic drill. There is risk to a listener's ears if loudness consistently exceeds 85 db (Fantal, 1990). A decrease in hearing ability can never be restored. Many earphone listeners and rock devotees have suffered measurable hearing loss.

YOU DON'T HEAR YOURSELF AS OTHERS HEAR YOU

Many singers feels that they must sing louder as they sing higher. This can be explained not only by the fact that you can't hear yourself as others hear you, but also by the fact that there is a muscle in your ear called the tensor tympani, which automatically decreases the mobility of the tympanic membrane when sounds become too loud. In other words, nature has given you protection against your own voice. When females sing high notes, they approach the area where the ear is most sensitive. This triggers the tensor tympani, giving you the illusion that your voice is too soft. People listening to you will tell you the opposite, that they can hear your voice very clearly. *Don't try to hear yourself!* It has been estimated that if the tensor tympani were not there, the sound inside your head could produce a tone as much as 20 db *above* the threshold of pain!

You hear your voice inside your head not only by air and tissue vibration, but by bone conduction as well. Chapter XVII on Neurology explains that there are sensory systems from your vocal folds and the tissues around your larynx that help you perceive what adjustments your voice is making in response to your thought of pitch. There are reflex interconnections between the sensory nervous supply to the larynx and the middle ear muscles (McCall, 1971). Add to this that you hear the sound of your voice by air conduction from the outside of your mouth to your ear and by acoustic feedback as the sounds you make reverberate off of walls, and the like. Both acoustic feedback and air conduction come too late to be of help. The sound has already left your body. You must sensitize yourself to the inner hearing— your proprioceptive sense of your voice.

EAR MUSCLES AND FATIGUE

Like all muscles, the muscles in your ear can get tired. If your ears are subjected to loud sounds too long, the sounds no longer seem loud; your sensitivity is dulled. This is why a symphony orchestra will build up to the climax of a piece by getting loud for only a short time and then dropping down to a softer level to start building up again. The longer your ear is exposed to an intense sound, the longer it will take to recover its former sensitivity. If not enough time is allowed, it will take longer to recover its sensitivity and greater intensity will be required to cause the ear to recognize a change in dynamics. Fatigue will be greater for more intense sounds, sounds that last longer, and sounds of higher frequencies. The high, loud screech of a fire siren or the loud take-off noise of an airplane are sometimes referred to as "deafening"—quite true, if you are exposed to them often enough.

Considerable body energy is expended each day in just resisting noise. If you want to have a truly restful vacation, seek a quiet place in the country. Going somewhere noisy might give you a change of scenery but it won't give you a rest. Not just your ears, but your whole body benefits from quiet surroundings.

Amplification in movie houses as well as theaters—especially Broadway musical theaters—has risen to such a level that it could be a threat to your hearing. If the trend continues, theater goers' hearing could be damaged to such a degree that overamplification becomes necessary for their enjoyment. Can you imagine what the buildup might lead to in 100 years? In the end, the promoters of louder and louder sound are defeating themselves. Why not devise ways to increase sensitivity instead of killing it? Urban noises, driving in a car, listening to a radio, phonograph, or television that is turned up too loudly (discos!!!) can all contribute to the fatigue or potential deterioration of the ear. Personally, I can't go to a movie or Broadway show without putting cotton or something protective in my ears. The same goes for flying in an airplane.

"Generally speaking, the vowels have higher intensities than the consonants" (Hirsch, 1952). Because consonants are necessary for intelligibility, they need to be exaggerated. Although consonants have less intensity, they are produced at higher frequencies. This is one reason that a person who has had a high frequency loss in his hearing finds it difficult to understand what is being said. As a performing artist, you must try to bring the intensity level of the consonants up to the level of the vowels.

It should be clear by now that the loudness of a note may change when the frequency (pitch) is changed, although the intensity (energy) remains the same. If you skip to a higher pitch with no change in energy, it will sound louder. Increasing or decreasing energy will, in itself, raise or lower a pitch, but it is better to change muscular adjustments than to use more energy to sing higher notes.

A very talented young student had a hearing deficiency in one ear. Although he had a full, strong voice, he kept complaining to me that he wanted to have more strength in his singing. Finally, he changed teachers and went to a man who had a reputation for building big voices. After being with the man for some time, he developed vocal polyps, which were subsequently removed through an operation. He had not trusted his sensations and what others told him they heard. He thought his career was over. Back home, he went to his former teacher, with whom he had a very friendly relation and eventually was able to resume his career. Not everyone is so lucky.

Sometimes the problem of flatting is related to starting a note with too much energy and then "pushing" it up to the desired frequency. If it is kept in mind that the pitch should be established in the muscles, there will be a sense of "starting tones from the top." Using the freedom of speech inflection will permit you to slide the pitch either up or down just by thinking. Matching your frequency to an accompaniment is extremely important.

A listener can sometimes experience what is known as *auditory fatigue*, a fact seldom considered by the performer. If a sound is being produced softly, the listener's ear will "reach out" to hear it. If the tone is too loud, the listener's ear will dampen to shut out part of the excessive sound. The idea is to let the listeners come to you. In working this idea, remember that there is such a thing as being too soft.

TROUBLE WITH PITCH—DIPLACUSIS

I had a student some years ago who would be exactly on pitch at times, and at other times would be very much off key. I frankly did not know what was going on and eventually the faculty felt that this student was in the wrong business. It was after that when I heard for the first time about a special hearing disorder.

I am indebted to Orin Cornett of Gallaudet College for information on a malfunction known as *diplacusis*. This is a condition in which a subject's two ears record different pitch sensations for the same tone. In 1954, Cornett hypothesized that diplacusis was a common cause of inability to sing on pitch. This has been confirmed in research by Culpepper (1957). A test for diplacusis could also be useful in identifying special problems such as a tendency to sing off pitch in only one small part of a scale. Testing for this difficulty can be done by a properly trained person, such as a hearing pathologist or an otolaryngologist, by using the Cornett diplacusimeter.

Singers and violinists in particular (musicians who do not use fixed pitch instruments like the piano and organ) can suffer greatly from this condition. There can be a late onset, a development of the complaint after one is well into one's career, in which case it can be catastrophic. Fortunately, something can be done about it in many cases.

If it is substantial, diplacusis can be detected by covering each ear alternatively while listening to a sustained tone. By using the Cornett diplacusimeter, discrepancies can be observed from a small fraction of a semitone to three semitones. In some subjects, the discrepancy approaches an octave!

The condition is often connected to allergic reaction to substances like coffee and chocolate and can be connected with Meniere's syndrome. In children, its effect can cause chords of music to sound confused, fuzzy, or even disagreeable. When such children listen with one ear, they appear to be able to do what a normal child does, learning easily to match pitch by tuning to eliminate the beat (generated in the ear) between one's voice and the reference tone. Presumably, because they do not develop this ability early in life, it often takes them longer to develop a memory for the musical scale and to match a tone after it has stopped without the benefit of the beat phenomenon. (The pulsations resulting from two tones of slightly different frequencies being sounded at the same time are called beats.)

This disability is apparently still not recognized in many schools of music, since I had never heard about it myself until I learned from Dr. Cornett. Testing should be done whenever a question of matching pitch presents itself.

PRESERVE YOUR HEARING

A complete physical exam is administered to all incoming students at the Royal Danish Conservatory of Music. All students must have a hearing test as well as a laryngeal examination. For the three-year course in opera training, often only three to five students are admitted each year. Although the course is not limited to Danes, students must have a working knowledge of the Danish language. Also, in this school, any student who is having vocal problems is referred to a voice therapist for weekly treatments, while continuing with his or her regular teacher. This is the most successful program I have encountered anywhere.

Teachers of singing should have a hearing test from time to time. I knew of one teacher who did not do this, and whose students seemed to keep singing louder and louder. Unfortunately, there is little anyone can do in such a situation unless the teacher himself asks for assistance or advice. This places great responsibility on students to exercise judgment and make a decision that will be in their own best interest.

Your hearing is a very important part of your equipment as a singer. Take good care of your ears and learn to respect how they can help you in gaining a good technique for your voice.

REFERENCES

Bartholomew, W. T. (1942). *Acoustics of music*, New York: Prentice Hall.

Culpepper. (1957). *Unpublished doctoral dissertation*, Nashville, Tn: Peabody College.

Culver, C. A. (1941). *Musical acoustics*, Philadelphia, Pa: The Blakiston Co., pub.

Fantal, H. (1990, March 18). *Listeners pay a high price for loud music*, New York Times, (p. 20).

Hirsh, I. J. (1952). *The measurement of hearing*, London: McGraw-Hill, (p. 126).

McCall, G. (1977). *Studies in spastic dysphonia, Projected research concerned with central neurologic pathologies on laryngeal dysfunction*, Transcripts of the 6th Symposium, Care of the professional voice, New York: The Voice Foundation (p. 91).

Zemlin, W. R. (1968). *Speech and hearing science*, Englewood Cliffs, NJ: Prentice-Hall.

XIX

■

ENIGMAS

Enigma: 1: an obscure speech or writing; 2: something hard to understand or explain; 3: an inscrutable or mysterious person.

Psychogenic: originating in the mind or in mental or emotional conflict—Merriam-Webster (1981).

"What's your hang-up?"

Do you know anyone who doesn't have or hasn't had problems at sometime or other? I've often wondered what it might be like if, when meeting someone at a social gathering, I were to ask him what his hang-up was.

No doubt you have known artists (not to mention relatives, friends, or associates) who faced crises that interrupted their work, or maybe even put an end to it. This can be especially true in the field of singing. Why? Think of what has been said from Chapter I on and you will know. In your nervous system, there is a direct connection between the vocal folds and the medulla oblongata, the nerve center for autonomic phonation.

PSYCHOGENIC EFFECTS ON SINGING

One year I worked with a student who had a promising voice but who did not progress in her first year at school as I had expected. In her second year, her voice began to take off and unfold as I had hoped it would the year before. I asked her what had happened during the summer to make such a big change. She replied that in her first year she had felt intimidated by the talented older students. During the summer, she decided that she was not going to let the effect of all these other students get to her. She was going to "do her stuff" and not bother about what anyone else was doing.

I often tell students the only competition that they have is themselves—the challenge to explore their own potential and to do justice to the music. This student was fortunate to have identified her bête noire and to have conquered it, but not everyone is so fortunate. At one point, I worked with a promising coloratura who had begun minor engagements amidst widespread praise for her skill and the beauty of her voice. At about this time, she announced that she had a new boyfriend who was devoted to her. He was married, but he was planning to divorce his wife. Not long afterwards, the man was transferred to the West Coast, but my student took comfort in the thought that it would be easier to get a divorce in Reno or in Mexico.

After some weeks, this student was not doing so well in her lessons, so I asked her what news she had had from her friend. She reported that there had been no letter or phone call—nothing. After three months, her singing was so bad that she left me, saying that I was ruining her voice. I later learned that she had worked with another teacher for a short time and then returned home and took a job in a restaurant.

It takes a lot of guts to face up to a situation like that, to call a cad a cad. Without the courage, the spirit suffers and so, usually, does the singing.

EFFECTS OF STRESS

Often you don't know what's hit you or why when something goes wrong. I once worked with a happily married young woman who had the time and resources to take up the study of singing, something she had always wanted to do. The resources came from her husband's professional success, but the reason she had time was not so fortunate. Her husband had been in an accident, was in a nursing home, and was unconscious a good deal of the time. This student was doing everything possible for her husband. She went to see him every day, and always took him something, even though he often did not recognize her. Finally, for self preservation she decided that she needed to occupy herself with something she would enjoy.

In beginning her lessons, my student seemed to be completely adjusted to her unfortunate circumstances. Her progress was remarkably good. She had played the piano previously, so she could work with songs very early in her study. Then one day she phoned to say she would not be in for her lesson because her husband had died, but to please save her time for the following week.

I went to the memorial service and found my student conservatively dressed and greeting friends much as if she were holding a reception. She had probably lived through the experience so often in her imagination that it was almost like acting out a part in a play. She greeted me with a smile, thanked me for coming, and said she would see me the following week.

Sure enough, she came for her lesson the next week, the week after, and the next one, and progressed beautifully. The fourth week, however, she came in looking very frustrated. "I've lost my voice," she said in a whisper. We talked about this. I explained how the emotions have a direct connection to the voice and also explained that she was going through one of the most traumatic experiences one can have, the loss of a spouse. I urged her to come the next week to follow up in the adjustment, which she did. In a few weeks her voice had returned to normal and so had her singing.

These three histories illustrate three different levels of stress. In a 1973 article for *The New York Times*, Jane E. Brody describes a "Scale of Impact Due to the Stress of Adjusting to Change" created by Thomas H. Holmes. Forty-three high-stress events are presented on a scale, with death of a spouse at 100%, or the most severe, and minor violations of the law at 11%, the opposite end of the scale. Changing schools is listed at 20% and marital separation registers at 65%. Brody states that "stress often precipitates physical as well as emotional illness . . . up to 80% of serious physical illnesses seem to develop at a time when the victims feel helpless and hopeless" (p. 20).

You can't fool Mother Nature! If you feel physically unwell or emotionally troubled, you'd better try to understand what is going on and do something about it. Your situation could become much worse if you don't.

If your difficulty is something you recognize, try putting it into one of three categories: (1) You know what the difficulty is and you realize that there is something you can do about it—do it; (2) You have identified the problem but do not believe this is the time to act—wait for the right opportunity and then take care of it; (3) You know what is wrong, you have thought about it from all angles, and see no solutions—adapt to your circumstances as best you can. If you can identify a problem, think it through; don't let it hang around your neck.

Of course, this is so easy to say and hard to do. Many problems do not fall into these simple categories. Often when you are disturbed, you can't imagine why. As Samuel Kraines wrote in 1948, "Fundamentally, man is not a rational animal. Man's reactions to his parents, to his family, to his pleasures, to his friends, to his association with others, to social organizations are far more dependent upon his 'feeling tone' than upon that which he reasons" (p. 21).

Without knowing the facts behind unusual behavior, how can you pretend that there is no reason why a voice does not respond? The subconscious effects of the mind on the voice can be very subtle. A book by Paul Moses (1954), entitled *The Voice of Neurosis*, gives fascinating insight into the interplay of the two.

At the subconscious level we are vulnerable to impulses derived from the so-called fight-or-flight response. Actions perceived as threats cause a sudden rise of adrenaline, and as Michael Hutchinson (1986) wrote in *Mega Brain*, "with blood and oxygen directed toward the muscles and away from the brain, the brain simply does not operate very well" (p. 89). Hutchinson also describes a study in which students under the greatest stress scored 13% lower during IQ tests than students under the least stress. For further discussion on the link between relaxation and superior performance, I refer you to Dr. Edmond Jacobson's (1952) book *Progressive Relaxation.*

In recent years, there has been much interest in biofeedback as a means of reducing stress. Biofeedback heightens your awareness of what's going on in your body and gives you voluntary control over so-called involuntary responses (Miller, 1983). *New Mind, New Body* by Barbara B. Brown (1974) presents the techniques of biofeedback in detail. In it, Brown states, "Biofeedback can provide the accurate, continuous indicators you need to know when and how your tension develops, and when and how it diminishes" (p. 8).

In March 1979, I presented a paper on laryngeal dysfunction at the International Symposium on the Larynx in San Francisco entitled "Treating the Fears of the Professional Voice User." To quote the famous English otolaryngologist Norman Punt, "Singers and actors are sensitive, excitable people readily influenced, a prey to their emotions, reacting violently to changes in environment" (1979, p. 1). I knew a singer of international reputation who was told after a performance that someone in the audience had casually said, "Well, his career didn't last long." It happened that the singer had performed while fighting a cold. The comment undermined his next performance, in spite of the fact that he knew perfectly well that he had made the best of a difficult situation and would be back to normal soon.

Professional singing is a fragile existence, requiring constant support and encouragement. Skill at self-governance is required to manage the small crises that will inevitably arise and the larger setbacks that may befall you as well. This is particularly true when traveling. Not all throat doctors know how to deal with professional artists. I had a student who was singing the lead role with an opera company in Italy. She felt she was coming down with a cold, but decided to sing that evening just the same. At the end of the first act, she asked the house physician to examine her throat. "Your vocal cords look like chopped meat," he told her. He then applied an aerosol spray of cortisone and prescribed cortisone injections three times a day, plus antibiotic injections three times a day for three days. She completed her performance that night, but canceled the next one. Not feeling any better four days later, she went to the head laryngologist at the local medical school. His remarks included the following: "You singers are always complaining about how sick you are. Your cords are not closing. In five years I'll bet you five to one that you'll have vocal nodules. I advise you to stop all medication immediately and to only take a new brand of aspirin put out by Bayer." In one and a half weeks, the singer, now in another city, checked with the phoniatric there who said, "Your vocal cords are O.K. Just gargle with hot water and salt."

Even if an infected throat look like raw beef, that's no way for a doctor to talk to the leading lady in the middle of a performance. Nor was the second opinion indicative of the proper attitude to encourage a young singer back to health. Good care is hard to find away from home. Fortunately these examinations were the exception, not the rule. The best defense is to keep a level head and to develop techniques for relaxing and keeping your emotions under control. You also have to know how to bring your voice back to performance level after a cold.

YOUR EMOTIONS CAN WORK FOR OR AGAINST YOU

Many emotional hang-ups come to light quite unexpectedly. A remark misunderstood or taken out of context may be imbued with significance that was never intended by the speaker.

At one time, I worked with a student who seemed to have nothing wrong with her voice, yet I felt she was holding back. She had range, but left the impression that there was something more, perhaps the potential for greater fullness on some notes. I asked about her home life as a child, and with seeming embarrassment she explained that her parents and other relatives were all very accomplished. I asked her if her family had expected a great deal from her when she was growing up, and she responded with great feeling that although she tried very hard, she never felt that she could satisfy her family with anything she did.

We experimented with a little exercise suggested by Eloise Ristad (1982) in her book, *A Soprano on Her Head.* We imagined that her relatives were sitting in different chairs around the room, and she was to tell them just what she thought of them. It was such fun. She began to laugh as she looked at them. They looked so human and helpless. Of course, this brought an immediate improvement in her singing.

Biofeedback, sympathy, empathy, stress, and emotional environment can all affect voice quality and control. The subtleties of fear in its many guises can wreak havoc with a singer's performance. A careless remark by a conductor or director can be most disturbing to a singer unless he or she has sufficient confidence to brush it aside and go ahead with what he or she feels is right.

I remember a student who was in rehearsal for the new production of very important opera revival. In the story, two ladies vie for the affection of a great king. The lady singing the part of the reigning queen was a famous leading artist. Her protagonist, my student, was told by the stage director to play down her role. She asked for a conference to discuss the interpretation because she felt that her part should be portrayed with strength, since in the end she would win the king's love. The director berated her in the presence of others for trying to be a prima donna, which caused her great frustration. Talking this over with me, I advised her to be cooperative in rehearsals but, in performance, to play the role exactly as she perceived it. The reviewer of the opening night declared that a proper protagonist had been found for the part, and the director rushed to her saying that she had done exactly what he wanted! "To thine own self be true, and it must follow, as the night the day, Thou canst not then be false to any man" (Shakespeare; *Hamlet*, Act I, scene iii).

Much has been written about the effect of emotions on body tensions and laryngeal adjustments. These studies go back to the time of the Greeks, and include the writings of Darwin and Freud. (Incidentally, I was told that Freud's first patient suffered from serious throat tension.)

If you let feelings in, your voice and your ability to control your voice will be affected. The danger lies in succumbing to emotions as you perform, rather than developing your theatrical abilities.

A great singer had been working very hard to improve her acting. In one very emotional scene, she began to shed real tears. "Ah, at last," she thought, "Now I really know how to act."

When she came off stage, the director took hold of her and shook her violently. "Don't you ever do that again," he yelled. Can you imagine what a basket case you would be if you gave yourself over to the emotions suggested in each piece of music you performed? Your job is to create the illusion of emotion so that the audience can cry. After all, you're there for them, not vice versa.

In his biography of *Maria Malibran* (1808–1836), Howard Bushnell (1979) relates an incident that took place in Bologna. The famous violinist Ole Bull was standing in the wings one night, and was so completely overcome by the ravishing voice and intense dramatic powers of Malibran's performance that tears ran down his face. Catching sight of him, Maria turned from the audience for a split second, gave him a ridiculous grimace, and was instantly back in character before an audience convinced she was living her role. On being confronted by Bull after the performance, Maria commented gaily, "It wouldn't do for both of us to blubber" (pp. 146–147).

Emotions affect your autonomic nervous system. This is why, under some stressful circumstances, a person will vomit. Friedrich Brodnitz relates a tale from his days as a student in Vienna. Late to the opera one evening and taking a shortcut through a side street, he encountered a man who was obviously sick to his stomach. Being a medical student at the time, Brodnitz asked if he could help. The man was the great tenor Leo Slezak (1873–1946), who replied, "No, thank you. I do this before every performance."

Feodor Chaliapin (1873–1938), considered by many as possibly the greatest singing actor that ever lived, needed to be constantly reassured that his voice sounded right and that the listeners liked what he was doing. He always had a young friend sit in the audience and come backstage as soon as he had finished his scene to report the audience's reaction.

Stage fright or performance anxiety is familiar to most who've gone before the public. The actress Gertrude Lawrence once said, "These attacks of nerves seem to grow more with the passing years. It's inexplicable and horrible and something you'd think you'd grow out of, not into" (Funk, 1982). Helen Hayes usually went stone deaf on opening nights. Mike Burstyn, star of the musical *Barnum*, says his stage fright results from the fear of audience rejection (Funk, 1982).

According to George A. Gates, (Performance Anxiety, 1992), "a sudden, severe, frightening or fearful stimulus causes the release of large amounts of catacholamines, resulting in perspiration and constriction of blood vessels (the cold clammies), a pounding or palpitating heart, dry mouth, muscle tension, and tremor (the shakes). At the same time, the parasympathetic system shuts down and digestion ceases, leading to a sense of gastric distress and even nausea. These symptoms are the classic 'fight or flight' response. When elicited by internally fearful stimulation such as internal conflict (Will I fail? Will I make a mistake? Will they not like me?), these same symptoms develop and are recognized as stage fright."

Regarding the use of beta blockers to combat stage fright, I'll share with you the following from a paper by George A. Gates and Phillip J. Montalbo (1987): "The effectiveness of B-Blocker use in singing students brought only slight improvement at low doses and a detrimental effect on performance at higher doses" (p. 105). Gates and Montalbo conclude that "a certain level of tension provides a sense of immediacy and life to performance that is desirable. We argue that their use (B-blockers) for singers is not justified by evidence accumulated to date" (p. 107).

Many people seek the advice of trained counselors to address the emotional problems that inhibit good performance. Singing teachers should not attempt to be psychiatrists! If there seems to be a need for help along these lines, I never say, "You ought to see a psychiatrist." Instead, I ask, "Do you think it would help you to have a professional evaluation?"

Psychological problems should be handled with the utmost tact and sensitivity. In the end, the thinking part of the singer's brain has to learn to control the emotional part. A singing teacher can encourage this mastery, but plumbing the depths of another's psyche is quite another matter. Kahlil Gibran's (1926) book *The Prophet* includes a chapter entitled "Reason and Passion." In this chapter, Gibran sums up what I feel an artist must do—"Let your soul exalt your reason to the height of passion that it may sing" (p. 45).

REFERENCES

Brody, J. E. (1973, June 10). *Doctors study tratment of ills brought on by stress*, The New York Times (p. 20).

Brown, B. B. (1974). *New mind, new body*, New York: Harper & Row, (p. 8).

Bushnell, H. (1979). *Maria Malibran*, University Park, Pa: Pennsylvania State University Press (pp. 146–147).

Funk, P. (1982). *Stage fright*, Stagebill, (p. 6).

Gates, G. A., & Montalbo, P. (1987). *The effect of low-dose B-blockade on performance anxiety in singers*, Journal of Voice, 1, New York: Raven Press (pp.105–108).

Gates, G. A.(1992). *Performance anxiety (stage fright); causes and control*, (Unpublished paper quoted with permission).

Gilbran, K. (1926). *The prophet*, New York: Knopf, (p. 45).

Hutchinson, M. (1986). *Mega brain*, New York: Beech Tree Books (p. 89).

Jacobson, E. (1952). *Progressive relaxation*, Chicago, Il: University of Chicago Press.

Kraines, S. H. (1948). *The therapy of the neuroses and psychoses*, Philadelphia: Lea and Febiger (p. 21).

Merriam-Webster. (1981). *Eighth new collegiate dictionary*, Springfield, Ma: Merriam-Webster.

Miller, L. (1983, June 6). *Stress: Can we cope?*, Quoted in Time, (p. 48).

Moses, P. (1954). *The voice of neuroses*, New York: Grune & Stratton.

Punt, N. A. (1979). *The singer's and actor's throat*, London: Heinemann (p. 1).

Ristad, E. (1982). *A soprano on her head*, Moab, Ut: Real People Press.

XX

■

Voice Problems And Therapy

I assume the prerogative to write this chapter based on my sixteen years of service as Lecturer in Voice Therapy at Washington University School of Medicine (1952–1968) and St. Louis City Hospital (1954–1968). Since that time I have kept up with this work through my private practice in New York City. However, I hasten to add that I have never seen a patient or singer in need of voice therapy who has not been examined by a throat specialist.

While I have no medical degree, and hence refrain from making medical diagnoses, I have worked with several thousand people in the role of voice therapist. When I started my work in St. Louis, I felt like a babe in the woods, but circumstances gave me confidence in approaching my task. First, I had direct experience with being taught bad vocal habits. My earliest training had led me to push, to do too much. Negative experiences some years later with so-called "experts" prompted me to explore how the voice really does function. On the positive side, my study with Arthur Wilson and my reading of books by H. Holbrook Curtis (1974) and Chevalier Jackson (Jackson & Jackson, 1937) gave me much of the background I needed to help those with voice difficulties. An opportunity to observe the work of David Blair McClosky in 1952 gave me assurance that I was on the right track, although we did some things quite differently. McClosky (1959) had been experimenting in therapy techniques with I. Blaisdel and D. W. Brewer in Syracuse since 1947.

In his book, Curtis gives an account of seeing a singing student with vocal nodules at about the same time that he saw another student with bowed vocal cords, each studying with different teachers. He recommended that the student with nodules study with the teacher of the student with bowed cords and vice versa. Each student corrected her condition and swore by her new teacher. This story illustrates a basic principle of voice therapy. Treatment seeks to eliminate the malfunction and replace it with healthy phonation. It is often a question of opposites.

Not many people know that Nellie Melba had vocal nodules just before and during her first visit to the United States. She kept this from the public all her life because she did not want to hurt the reputation of her teacher, Matilda Marchesi.

Soon after Melba arrived in the United States, she experienced some vocal difficulty and consulted Dr. Curtis, a specialist who treated all the great singers of her era. When he told her she had vocal nodules she replied, "Impossible!" After some questioning, she confessed that she had experienced some difficulty in the previous year in England and that Sir Morrill McKenzie advised her to take a rest, suggesting that she had become overtired. Curtis asked if he might contact McKenzie to ask him what his diagnosis had been. McKenzie replied, "Vocal nodules," and added that he did not tell Mme. Melba his finding because he did not want to frighten her. Learning this, Curtis prescribed some voice exercises for Melba to rehabilitate her voice. She followed his routine faithfully, regained her vocal health, and maintained it for the rest of her long career. The fact that Curtis prescribed corrective exercises indicates that Melba's difficulties were functional, that is, she was misusing her voice muscles.

FUNCTIONAL DISORDERS

In his book *Vocal Rehabilitation*, Friederich Brodnitz (1959) describes two types of functional disorders: hyperfunction (too much) and hypofunction (too little), with by far the greater number of cases falling in the first category. In this chapter, I will review the basic causes of hyper- and hypomalfunction disorders and attempt to describe how each is of particular concern to singers. Although any one malfunction (improper use) can cause a voice disorder, often several of them combine to produce the first conspicuous signs of trouble.

Although 95% of cases referred to me in St. Louis concerned the speaking voice, I learned early on what is healthy for the speaking voice is also healthy for singing.

Almost all professional voice users seek the guidance of a speech or singing teacher at one time or another. Hopefully, those who guide these people keep the following points in mind:

1. Speech and singing are human inventions.
2. Each person brings his or her own set of physical equipment and his or her own potential to the "art" of making sound.
3. Since voice use and training are athletic endeavors, the laws of growth (maturation) and muscular development should be observed.
4. Because vocal expression is linked to emotional expression, the psyche can play an important role in the entire pattern of voice use.
5. Urban living, noisy environment, the telephone, and the like place greater stress on the voice than was true 100 years ago, yet our bodies have not undergone a physiological change to compensate for it.

Those who depend on their voices for their livelihood must endeavor to maintain their health with the same seriousness as a professional athlete. (Remember, vocalizing is an athletic activity.) This means maintaining a proper diet and getting regular rest and exercise. It also means avoiding overuse of the voice. Oddly enough, even among singers it is often excessive talking (not singing) which leads to difficulty. Speaking and singing rely on the same phonatory muscles.

I once asked a new patient whether she felt she talked a lot. She said she felt she talked no more than the average person, although I had difficulty conducting the conference because she talked so continuously. Quite by coincidence, my next patient was an acquaintance of hers. After the first patient left, the second commented, "Well! I'm not surprised to see her in your office. I never met anyone in my life who talks as much as she does!"

If you sing or speak professionally, I would discourage you from attempting to diagnose your own voice difficulties. If you run into a problem, consult a physician, preferably one aquainted with the types of difficulties professional voice users encounter. What can be seen by way of physical mannerisms or what is heard in voice quality is important to note. It would be valuable also to keep a log of any voice training or treatment you receive over the years; most medical examinations begin with a lengthy series of questions on medical history. If corrective exercises are recommended, or appear to be in order, they should be undertaken with the guidance of a licensed therapist or a teacher aquainted with the singing voice and educated in anatomy and physiology.

Some singing teachers have reputations of not forcing voices and of having a sensitive ear as to what constitutes healthy sound. On the other hand, there are therapists who have not had training in the singing voice who would be of very little assistance.

In 1992, the National Association of Teachers of Singing and the American Speech and Hearing Association issued a Joint Statement on "The Role of the Speech-Language Pathologist and Teacher of Singing in Remediation of Singers and Voice Disorders." This statement was published in the November/December 1992 issue of the *NATS* Journal, and the January 1993 issue of *ASHA*. The statement affirms "the importance of interdisciplinary management of singers with voice disorders, with the management team ideally consisting of, but not restricted to, at least an otolaryngologist, a speech-language pathologist and a singing teacher" (*NATS* Journal, p. 14).

Hyperfunction (Too Much)

The following is a list of 18 conditions that should be kept in mind in evaluating phonatory disorders. I have observed these conditions in singers of all ages and in all stages of study from beginners to professionals. The list is not definitive, but it covers the major causes of these phonatory disorders.

1. *Singing too loudly.* This can start with a mistaken idea of what it takes to sing. It can be a misconception of expressing feeling. It can also be from a desire to hear your own voice. (See Chapters VIII and IX.)
2. *Using the voice too long.* Phonatory muscles can fatigue like any other muscles. When your voice seems to be going well, there may be temptation to indulge in prolonged use, but you pay for it the next day.
3. *Pushing with the breath.* Many singers have the mistaken belief that increased effort from the lungs will help to strengthen the voice. (See Chapter VIII.)
4. *Straining for high notes.* Some singers feel that because they do not know what else to do for high notes that a greater effort will help. They compare singing high notes to reaching the top shelf in the pantry for a cookie. (See Chapter V.)

5. *Squeezing for low notes.* Low notes seem similar to grunting noises, and some singers use the push needed for a grunt to reach low tones. (See Chapter V.)

6. *Tension in the shoulders.* In extremes of breathing, the shoulders come into play and this is brought into singing, often unconsciously, with a false notion that the added action is needed for sound. (See Chapters III and IV.)

7. *Posture too rigid.* In an effort to stand straight, muscles for an erect body position are stiffened. This inhibits free breathing and tends to tighten neck muscles. (See Chapters II and III.)

8. *Breathing too high.* The instructions to "fill your lungs, throw out your chest, pull in your gut," can all lead to excessively high chest activity. Again, the resulting tension will transmit to the throat. (See Chapter III.)

9. *Breathing too low.* "Breathe low" is misunderstood as distending the lower abdominal area (as if the air could go down there!?). An inadequate supply of oxygen results, as well as an excessive pull on the larynx. (See Chapter III.)

10. *Tension in neck muscles.* In trying too hard, extrinsic neck muscles are brought into play that falsely mix with the larynx to produce sound. For free interplay of the intrinsic muscles, the extrinsic muscles must relax. (See Chapters II, III, and XVI.)

11. *Tension in muscles of articulation (tongue, lips, and jaw).* Realizing that more has to be done than in ordinary speech to be clearly understood, excessive attempts are made and overarticulation results. Articulation and phonation are independent but simultaneous. (See Chapters X and XVII.)

12. *Distortion of facial muscles.* Concentration and mental conceptions of hard work may be reflected in facial contortions, much as a child learning to write will move his mouth and cheeks, squint his eyes and raise his eyebrows. Such contortions (although they are entertaining) can inhibit free laryngeal adjustments. (See Chapter XVII.)

13. *Carrying low voice too high.* Singers are acquainted with their speaking quality and may mistakenly identify this as their whole voice. Doing so does not allow the cricothyroid muscles to assist in the adjustment for higher notes. (See Chapter V.)

14. *Too much overall use of voice, including speech.* Singers often forget that in speaking they are using the same muscles for phonation as for singing and therefore often bring tired muscles to their singing. (See Chapters IX and XVI.)

15. *Faulty speaking habits.* Singing uses language. If there have been problems with any aspects of speech, they will show up in singing. Often people speak higher or lower than is most efficient. Healthy habits are needed for both speaking and singing. (See Chapters IV and X.)

16. *Imitation of poor voice models.* Subconsciously you may imitate a relative, teacher or friend or a voice on radio, TV, or records that is not being used in a healthy manner. Find your own voice; it will serve you best. (See Chapter IV.)

17. *Trying for too much sound with young voices.* The throats of children and teenagers are not of sufficient size to make the same pitch adjustments or to produce the full resonance of a mature voice. (See Chapter VI.)

18. *Trying to sing difficult music before technically ready.* This would be much like an athlete trying to see how far he could throw the discus before he had learned how to hold it. Yet it happens all the time because a student likes a particular aria or song. Match repertoire to vocal development. (See Chapters IX and XII.)

Hypofunction (Too Little)

Hypofunction is not encountered so often. It is characterized by a breathy quality or what might be called a lack of energy in the voice. Air energy is not being transferred into acoustic energy. A breathy quality is natural in young voices, but when it continues into the mid-twenties or beyond, a thorough examination is indicated. If the larynx appears normal (except possibly for so-called bowed vocal folds), you can proceed with corrective exercise. Here are some examples of hypofunction:

1. *Not enough breath to finish normal phrases.* The sound can seem quite acceptable, yet it is necessary to take breaths too often. Sometimes a singer will even breathe in the middle of a word. (See Chapters III and IX.)

2. *Tone lacks carrying power.* There is a definite lack of resonance in the voice. No amount of effort seems to have any effect. Avoid pushing as a substitute. (See Chapter VIII.)

3. *The breathy quality can actually be heard—almost like whispering.* This quality can be heard in all parts of the

range and characterizes the entire voice production. In undeveloped adult and children's voices, some of this is natural. (See Chapters IV and IX.)

4. *Notes give out in the middle of the range.* At the lower end of Register 3 or upper range of Register 2, the blend of the two is not working. This can be the result of carrying a low voice too high. (See "mezza di voce" in Chapter IX.)

5. *Excessive breathiness in high tones.* This indicates that Register 3 has not been properly exercised. It deserves extra time and attention because the high voice is not used outside of singing. (See Chapter V.)

6. *Excessive breathiness in low tones.* This indicates a lack of association between the speaking voice and resonance with pitches. This can be the result of pushing down. (See Chapter V.)

7. *Loss of air in consonants.* The words seem to be made up primarily of vowels with little audible energy in consonants. This contributes to loss of air for extended phrases and results in very poor diction. Consonants need to be firm and crisp. (See Chapter X.)

8. *Psychological factors.* There are times when a voice will take on a breathy quality due to emotional distress or melancholy. These conditions need to be handled with the greatest of sensitivity and support, avoiding negative suggestions of any kind. Seek professional counseling for an evaluation of this condition. (See Chapter XIX.)

FURTHER EFFECTS OF FUNCTIONAL DISORDERS

Laryngitis

When carried to excess, hyper- or hypofunctions can lead to functional pathologies. The most common of these is what is known as *chronic laryngitis.* The individual sounds as though he had a cold, got over it, but hung on to the compensatory voice until it became a habit. Resting the voice does not change habits of phonation, although resting the voice to avoid forcing bad habits is recommended.

Edema, Polyps, and Nodules

When not corrected, chronic laryngitis can lead to edema, polyps, or vocal nodules. An *edema* is a swelling of the tissues covering the surface of the vocal folds due to retention of excess fluids. When this is localized in one area, a larger swelling filled with fluid can form what is known as a *polyp*. A *nodule* is a smaller but firmer swelling and can be unilateral or bilateral—on one or both vocal folds. Polyps and nodules can be compared to blisters or corns formed on your foot where there has been pressure and rubbing. If you stop wearing the shoe that is causing the irritation, it will go away. But when you start wearing the shoe again the problem will return. In the same way, voice rest will often allow the folds to become clear and smooth. Once you start talking with the old habit, however, the swelling returns. This is why exercises to change the functional habits help where no amount of medication or voice rest will produce a permanent cure. Surgery without therapy also is no guarantee. Lucrecia Bori (1887–1960) and Leo Slezak (1873–1946) both suffered vocal nodules. When they rested and then retrained their voices, they were able to continue singing for many years—Slezak into his seventies.

I once worked with a young lady who was employed by the telephone company while she studied singing. She talked all day long at her job interviewing customers. When she came down with a severe cold and laryngitis, she continued working. Her family doctor gave her a shot of penicillin. A week later, not showing any signs of recovery, she saw her family doctor again and he gave her more penicillin. After another week, still suffering from laryngitis, she returned to the doctor once more. This time he told her to see a throat specialist because he had given her enough penicillin for a horse!

The throat specialist told her she had vocal polyps which would need to be removed surgically. One week after the operation, having been on complete voice rest, she returned for a checkup. The specialist told her that everything looked absolutely normal and that she could resume speaking. She thanked him in a very rough voice. The doctor told her she should not use her voice in that way, and sent her to me. The operation had removed the polyps, but not the habit that produced them. Had therapy not been prescribed, the polyps would have returned.

The exercises described in Chapters II, IV, and V will produce changes in production if fitted to the needs of the individual. Remember that no two cases are exactly alike; where one patient might respond with the nodules, for example, being cleared in a matter of days, another might require six to eight weeks of therapy scheduled twice a week. The number of treatments received depends on the extent of damage to be repaired and the patient's willingness to experiment with and adapt to new strategies for making sound.

The value of voice therapy in treating nodules was clearly demonstrated to me during my days at Washington University Medical School. There, I treated a man who worked as a foreman in a noisy factory. He had had vocal nodules surgically removed 42 times, but following voice therapy, there were no recurrences.

Dysphonia Plicae Ventricularis

A condition called dysphonia plicae ventricularis means phonating with the ventricular bands—the "false vocal cords." This is caused by extreme hyperfunction. The vocal folds are pressed so hard that they can do no more, so the muscles above the folds get into the act. This condition can be caused by using the voice when lifting heavy objects. Singers can approach this type of hyperfunction in pressed singing. When the folds themselves do not seem to produce the desired sound, the singer resorts to excessive effort, creating a grunting sound. The treatment, of course, is to establish a relaxed throat and neck and easy breathing with light breathy exercises. (See Chapters II and IV.)

Contact Ulcers

Contact granuloma, or contact ulcers as it is sometimes called, is also associated with hyperfunction. The larynx usually rests a little on the high side and the phonation tends to be constrained. Tension reduction exercises with special attention on letting the larynx rest in a low position are needed. The exercises for eliciting phonation, but without pitches, can be started as indicated in Chapter IV.

A famous popular singer referred to me with this condition reworked his entire repertoire with his "new voice" before starting work again. I saw him next some five years later performing in a night club in San Francisco. He told me he hadn't had a night off since resuming work!

Myasthenia Larynis

A college voice teacher once came to me with a condition much like *myasthenia laryngis*, laryngeal muscles much strained from overuse. Her condition had advanced to such a degree that she could barely speak enough to instruct her students, let alone sing.

It took the better part of a year to rehabilitate her voice, first her speech and then her singing. At the end of that time, she sang in a recital at her school and everyone agreed that it was the best singing she had ever done. Only by the most careful discipline was she able to sustain her new voice, but it served her through the remainder of her teaching years.

Myasthenia laryngis can be difficult to diagnose. Symptoms of vocal fatigue at the end of the day or the end of a week of regular voice use can be a danger signal. Often it is not recognized until it has gone too far. This subject has been thoroughly described in Jackson's book, *The Larynx and its Diseases* (Jackson & Jackson, 1937). To avoid myasthenia laryngis or similar conditions, follow the example of the great bass Feodor Chaliapin (1873–1938), who said that he always tried to perform with a reserve, knowing that he could sing louder if he wanted to. Chaliapin had a very long career.

Designing Treatment for the Individual

Over the years I've learned that every voice problem (treatable through therapy) requires its own course of action and its own schedule of treatments. There are no set rules. A student's progress indicates the next step in therapy. Treatments, quite literally, must be "played by ear."

To facilitate vocal reeducation, I ask my students to speak no more than absolutely necessary during the course of the corrective treatments, and never loudly. The sessions usually start with tension reduction exercises and attention to easy, natural breathing. This sometimes is all that is accomplished in the first meeting. Next, we experiment with single sighing sounds to find the ones that are easiest. Often there will be only a few sounds that flow easily. These are then practiced ten times each at each practice. I recommend practice six times a day with at least an hour between. Ten minutes is usually enough for the complete practice session. Never hurry to get through the exercises. Sometimes little bits can be done at odd moments. I worked with one man with vocal polyps who was a very busy executive and over 70 years of age. He made excellent progress. I was amazed and asked him how long he practiced. He answered, "Six times a day for ten minutes each. That's what you told me, wasn't it? I have my secretary put it down in my appointment calendar and see no one and receive no phone calls during that time." No wonder he made such good progress and got rid of his polyps! He treated his practice as though it were any other piece of business, and he didn't want an operation! I saw him fewer than ten times for treatments but a letter from the doctor who referred him, Dr. Walsh, testifies that the polyps disappeared.

As improvement shows, gradually more sounds can be added. When it is evident that half a dozen sounds are going easily, I have the person add counting in a lazy, slow, sing-song manner, in groups of 5 up to 50. That totals ten easy breaths. In another few days, short sentences can be added. The counting and sentences form the bridge over from easy sounds to easy speech. Without this, people comment that they can do the exercises but can't talk that way. A definite adjustment needs to be made to the "new voice." Finally, short periods of reading poetry, the newspaper, and so on can be added to feel the flow of the voice in communication.

Treatment for Hypofunction

The treatment for hypofunction is to correct breathy phonation. Staccato exercises are of value, provided they are done lightly to avoid the opposite extreme—hyperfunction. Commencing vowels with voiced consonants such as [b] and [d] is helpful. They can be alternated in speech. For example, say, "*Bi* di bi di *Bi*," "*Go* do go do *Go*," and so on, accenting the first and last sounds. Combining this with a light snapping motion of your forearm on the first and last syllables, as if shaking off some water, will help the adductor (closing) action. Find the combinations of consonant and vowel that produce the best phonation and repeat in short sessions each day. This exercise was shown to me by Svend Smith, who had great success with hypofunction cases.

Treatment for Cord Paralysis

Unilateral or bilateral cord paralysis should be treated with the assistance of a trained voice therapist. The so-called "pushing exercises" are of particular value but should not be over-done. Another way of inducing the folds to close is to practice a very light cough—as if lightly clearing your throat. An exercise I call the "dripping faucet exercise" is done by thinking a light, whispered glottal attack: [hə, ə, ə, ɚ-]. Try imitating a laughing reflex the same way, this time lightly phonated; only let the sounds be faster. Then try to sustain the last sound. Count in staccato rhythms, separating each number.

Ruptured Vocal Folds

Ruptured vocal folds occur very rarely. However, should you encounter such a condition, this case history should be of interest.

A student phoned at about 9:30 one evening barely able to talk. She said she had been attacked while bicycling on a vacant road. Her attacker had grabbed her tightly around the throat with his arm. She had struggled and screamed, but finally stopped and said, "What do you want?" "Your money," was the reply. "This is all I have, take it," she said, emptying her purse of about ten dollars. He took the money and ran away. She brushed herself off, examined her bruises and went home, noticing that she had practically lost her voice.

Although it was late when she called, I asked her to meet me at my studio as soon as she could. This was a Thursday night and she was scheduled to open as leading lady in a musical the following Tuesday.

I examined her larynx at the studio and saw that a blood vessel on her right vocal fold had ruptured. The whole larynx appeared very red and swollen. I did not tell her about the rupture, but merely said that her vocal cords were red and swollen.

It was too late to consult an otolaryngologist, so I put her on complete voice rest, gave her relaxing exercises and suggested she apply cold compress to her neck, take a sleeping pill, rest as well as possible and see me the next morning.

At the doctor's office the next morning I was amazed at how much less red her larynx looked and how much the swelling had reduced. She had a rehearsal, and I told her to walk through her part, silently shaping her words and to return to see me after rehearsal.

She came at about 5 p.m. Her throat looked better than it had in the morning; the rupture had reduced to a small swollen blood vessel.

I consulted with the doctor in the meantime and he told me to continue as I was; there was nothing he could do. That afternoon, I started her on the very lightest exercises to be done for one to two minutes each hour in addition to the relaxation routine.

She came to see me early Saturday morning. Again there was vast improvement. Most of the swelling had disappeared and the blood vessel was only a thin line. I asked her to continue on voice rest through rehearsal that day and to see me again at 5 p.m. By late afternoon all trace of the ruptured vessel had disappeared, although her vocal cords were still not normal in color. We increased the voice exercises to three to four minutes, and continued to do them very lightly.

By Sunday morning the swelling seemed entirely gone and the color was improved. For dress rehearsal I told this woman she could speak all of her lines softly but not sing her songs. (It was an open rehearsal and the accompanist said he made his debut as a singer doing her solos!) That afternoon, we went through her solos with a light, breathy voice.

Monday night was a public preview with no rehearsal during the day. She came for a lesson and her voice seemed to have some resonance, albeit soft. I told her to sing the performance that night exactly the same way. She reported Tuesday that it had gone beautifully and that she felt prepared for opening night. I instructed her to sing opening night the same way.

Success! She didn't use full voice but her songs "got across." The second night she was overconfident and sang a bit too loudly, which caused a slight setback. She returned to a conservative approach, however, and was able to continue through the run of the show, about three weeks.

Had she not been a highly self-disciplined person, this would not have been possible. She had been studying with me for several years before the incident, however, and had confidence in my instructions. Also, knowing my approach to singing, she knew how to practice exactly as I had directed. It was an extremely lucky outcome.

Childlike Voice After Puberty

Occasionally, one will encounter cases of incomplete mutation where a child's voice quality is carried beyond puberty. This often happens in families where there is a dominant mother and weak father. Mother wants to keep her darling little boy around as long as possible. In some cases, the only siblings are sisters.

Treatment is relatively simple. With strong, reassuring support, ask the boy to relax his head, jaw, and neck and then clear his throat gently, with the larynx in a relatively low position. Carry this into a voiced "uh huh."

After finding the "new" voice, reinforce it by repeating "Guh Guh Guh." Then try phrases like, "Oh No!" Experimenting with low, relaxed sounds will soon give the boy the assurance that he has a new voice he can use. Add counting in groups of five slowly, thus carrying phonation into speech. Assure him that it will take a little practice to firmly establish this new voice, but praise him for his discovery! It should take only one, two, or three sessions to establish the new voice.

This condition is usually manifest at ages 15 or 16, a time when the changed voice should have asserted itself. The most extreme case I ever had was a young man aged 28 who had just come out of the army where he held the rank of sergeant. He wanted to become a radio announcer, but obviously, something needed to be done about his voice. He was a married man with children and his voice sounded more like a high squeak than a man or woman. By following the same routine as that used with teenagers, he discovered his new voice and had it well established within a few weeks. (I don't know whether he ever got the job he wanted.)

Surgery

Many vocal fold pathologies—hematoma, hyperkeratosis, papilloma, leukoplacia, amyloid tumor, angioms and fibromata are examples—require surgery and post-operative voice therapy. Compensatory habits acquired before these conditions are treated cannot be corrected by surgery or voice rest. A follow-up of voice therapy is indicated.

A tonsillectomy is not dangerous to the voice if it is done by a competent surgeon. (The pillars of the fauci should not be clipped.) A patient may experience soreness from trauma in the surrounding muscle areas but with rest, it goes away. The voice may feel different afterward, but it will sound the same to others.

A deviated septum is a variance in bone structure in the nose. It can influence airflow in the nose and cause excessive dryness in the throat. Surgery for this does not affect the vocal folds. A singer might have to accustom him- or herself to new resonance sensations, but to others, there is usually no noticeable change in voice quality.

Nasal Resonance and Nasality

When your mouth is closed, the soft palate is dropped so that you can breathe through your nose. This position is necessary for the humming sounds m [m], n [n] and ng [ŋ] in the English language. *Nasality* results when the soft palate stays open in the production of vowel sounds. Some individuals need to strengthen the palatopharyngeus muscle, which elevates the soft palate. Individuals often do not know they have this problem because they are accustomed to the quality that a low soft palate creates.

A simple test is to read one sentence that has no nasal sounds in it while pinching your nostrils, and then a second sentence containing nasals. For example: "I feel as if we will have blue skies today," and "Don't dangle that mess in front of me." If nasal sounds are heard in the first sentence, there is nasality. The second sentence can't be read without nasals. Another way of testing is to blow bubbles through a straw into a glass of water. While doing this, pinch your nostrils. If more bubbles are blown when the nostrils are pinched, the soft palate is weak.

One exercise to help strengthen the soft palate is to blow up balloons. Another is to vigorously use such initial consonants as b, p, d, t, s, z, f, and v before vowels. For example, *bo, po, do, toe.* Be inventive. It takes time, but the problem can be treated.

Hoarseness

Jackson and Jackson (1937) list 60 diseases associated with hoarseness in adults and 35 in children. The beginnings of a laryngeal malfunction can be elusive. Sometimes, a child is born with an abnormal condition or acquires it very young. If a child has a "croupy" cold when learning to talk, that rough sound can be associated with speech although it doesn't belong there naturally. These conditions can be corrected by a trained therapist.

Other Considerations That Affect Voice

Much has been written about the need to keep the vocal folds adequately lubricated. This means creating or favoring environments with sufficient moisture. This can be particularly difficult in northern climates where heating tends to dry the air. Use a humidifier in areas where you spend the most time. In hotel rooms or at home, run the hot water in the shower very slowly while dressing or preparing for bed in the evening. This provides a helpful amount of moisture. Some people keep a supply of lemon drops or gum handy. You may have a favorite—without sugar!

Breathing through your nose is one of the best habits you can form in this regard.

Traveling

Be aware that humidity is very low in airplanes. A long flight can create a dry condition in your throat. Drink lots of water! Circulating water through your system helps eliminate waste and keep body tissues moist. The vocal folds need lots of moisture. The average person swallows as much as two quarts of mucous a day, according to research done some years ago by the late Dr. Doris Woolsey.

Air travel is also hard on the body and therefore the voice. When traveling long distances eastward, try eating and sleeping earlier for a couple of days before you leave. The opposite is true when traveling westward. If you have an ear infection, travel only with the advice of a doctor. Allow a free day for adjustment to the new time schedule after your arrival.

Menstrual Cycle

The female's menstrual cycle affects vocal function but will vary with individuals. The larynx will look different during menses. Changes may include excess fluid retention, a tendency toward hemorrhages on the vocal folds, and excess mucous. This may result in a slight decrease in the quality of high tones and flatness at the register changes and on high notes. Each singer must know her own menstrual adjustments if she is to avoid building compensatory habits. Many European houses provide female artists with free days for the menstrual cycle.

Pregnancy and Menopause

A pregnant woman may experience breathing problems during the last months and shortly after delivery. Menopause may result in a temporary or even permanent lowering of the voice or loss of the top notes. The voice may become wobbly, brittle, tremulous and perhaps weak. I have found that daily light vocalizing, especially exercising the light, upper part of the voice, helps to circumvent the difficulties than can come on at menopause. There are many examples of female artists who have sung well into their sixties and beyond. Magda Olivero made her debut at the Met as Tosca at age 67. I heard it. She was great!

Smoking

In this day, we all know what smoking can do to us, but some continue to smoke despite the obvious danger to themselves and others around them.

Let's consider the costs of smoking with respect to healthy voice use. Deposits left on the laryngeal and bronchial tissues, irritate. This results in coughing, which creates further irritation.

Smoking can damage the action of the epithelium (the covering of the vocal folds), which must be healthy for free vibration.

I saw many unfortunate results of smoking during my years of clinical work in St. Louis. Once, a voice teacher visiting there from another part of the country asked if he could observe my work. I had some particularly difficult cases that day. Some of the patients had had surgery for cancer of the tongue or mouth from smoking. I knew the teacher was a smoker, but I had no part in planning the list of patients I was to see that day. Some years later when I met him at a convention, he told me that he had quit smoking the very day of his visit and had not touched a cigarette since.

Prescription Drugs

Many drugs are harmful to the voice. A compendium of information on the effects of drugs and many other substances on the voice is available in *Professional Voice: The Science and Art of Clinical Care*, by Robert T. Sataloff (1991).

Cortisone should be avoided if possible and only taken under a doctor's guidance. Aspirin enlarges the blood vessels as do birth control pills. Aspirin should not be used to relieve fatigue before a performance. Because aspirin causes swelling of the blood vessels, it can be a predisposing factor to vocal fold hemorrhage. Birth control pills have been greatly refined but should always be taken in consultation with a doctor.

Alcohol

Alcohol relaxes muscles and swells the mucous lining in the throat. One's ability to monitor the voice is greatly reduced. A single cocktail will affect the voice for five hours. Caffeine in coffee, tea, or chocolate affects the nervous system and the voice.

Trauma From Accident

Trauma to the larynx from an accident can result in forced phonation, especially if the victim begins speaking too soon after the trauma. It is best to keep silent until the trauma to the larynx has been thoroughly diagnosed and then to begin talking very softly a little at a time.

Allergies

Allergies are particularly troublesome and have caused some fine artists to give up their careers. (To say the least, it's difficult to build a career when you have to schedule appearances around allergy season.) Anything affecting the mucosa, which lines the nose, mouth and pharynx, can also affect the larynx. That same lining extends down and covers the vocal folds. A good allergist can often treat these conditions so that a singer can cope with them. The treatment for allergy to cats, dogs, and so on, is obvious. Stay away from them.

Healthy Voice Use

To end this chapter on a positive note, let me try to describe what I mean by healthy voice use. If you can finish a performance feeling as though you could do it all over again, that's healthy. If you can sing several nights in a row and still feel comfortable singing the next day, that's healthy. If you can sing your high notes, low notes, loud notes, and soft notes and have them all clear with no evidence of push or strain, that's healthy. If you feel physically tired but can warm up your voice so it sounds fresh, that's healthy. If you know your physical condition is not normal, that you do not have sufficient energy to perform either because of a cold, a threatening cold, or physical fatigue and you cancel, that's healthy.

If you are teaching school five days a week and have been doing so for a number of years without getting hoarse or husky, that's healthy. If you are a salesman or minister and have a fresh, clear voice day after day, year after year, that's healthy. If you are a public speaker or actor making many speeches each week and always have a fresh, strong voice quality, that's healthy. If you speak in crowded, noisy places or if your work requires you to talk all day and your voice stays clear and strong, that's healthy.

Never compensate. It is better to do too little than to do too much. Remember that the voice responds to the mental concept.

THINK   LET   TRUST

REFERENCES

Brodnitz, F.S. (1959). *Vocal rehabilitation*, American Academy of Opthalmology and Otolaryngology, a Manual, Rochester, Mn: Whiting Press.

Curtis, H.H. (1974). *Voice building and tone placement*, Minneapolis, Mn: Pro Musica Press. (Reprint from New York: Appleton, 1896)

Jackson, C., & Jackson, C. L. (1937). *The larynx and its diseases*, Philadelphia, Pa: Saunders.

McClosky, D.B. (1959). *Your voice at its best*, Boston, Ma: Little, Brown.

NATS Journal. (1992, November / December). *The role of the speech-language pathologist and teacher of singing in remediation of singers with voice disorders*, (p. 14).

Sataloff, R. T. (1991). *Professional voice: the science and art of clinical care*, New York: Raven Press.

XXI

■

HINTS FOR TEACHERS

"**I** know you believe you understand what you think I said, but I am not sure you realize that what you heard is not what I meant."

Some years ago, a student gave me a little plaque with this quotation on it. I don't know who said it, but I keep it in a conspicuous place in my studio. It is comparable to a statement I often make in my lectures, namely that there is probably nothing that has ever been said or written about singing that cannot be misinterpreted.

I keep learning from my students. When I think I know exactly how to suggest something and it fails to produce the intended result, I'm reminded how feeble language can be.

I once explained to a student exactly how she should do a certain phrase and she sang it beautifully. To implant the experience in her memory, I said, "Good. Now tell me how you did it." She replied, "I felt I was doing exactly the opposite of what you told me to do!" How can we help but have moments like this?

EACH STUDENT IS DIFFERENT

This is the great challenge in teaching. And every student is different. To get the results I want, I often have to find new ways of instructing. For example, if I ask a student to feel the beginning of a yawn because pharyngeal space is needed and the student has previously been told to keep his larynx low, the result may be a woolly sound with the larynx much too low. In this circumstance,

235

I suggest to the student that he think of his soft palate as being quite high. The result is often what I want because a reflex action causes the larynx to drop when the soft palate is lifted.

Sensations are such an individual experience. What seems like "down and back" to one student will seem like "high and forward" to another.

I once had a student who would come in each week and explain the new sensations she was feeling. One time she would describe feeling as if the tone were coming out of the top of her head. Another time she would feel it at the back of her throat. Then she would say she felt as if there were a tin can on top of her head resonating the tone. Another time she would have the sensation that her voice was coming out of her ears. I told her she was the most "sensational" student I'd ever had!

This story shows how deceptive sensations can be. And, as a student progresses, sensations will change. That is why many fine performers who have discovered a sensation that seems to be present when they are singing their best do not necessarily make the best teachers. They know what they feel, but it may be difficult to explain to another singer.

I knew a teacher who had a strong, resonant voice which, he told me, he had had all his life. Unfortunately, many of his students suffered because he wanted to hear the same kind of sound from them. That's impossible! No two voices start from the same point.

I was told by a student who had studied with Toti dal Monti that when she asked how she, too, could learn to sing high notes, dal Monti replied, "It's a gift from God!" By using the techniques I described for finding the "flute voice," this student learned that she, too, could sing those high notes.

Many great artists are born with an instinct for what they need to do. It is easy to understand why they have difficulty empathizing with students starting with lesser skills or with problems they have never had to face. I've heard of a "teacher" in Italy who simply barked, "No!" when his students failed to execute a phrase properly, and "Si!" when they got it right.

UNDERSTANDING THE MECHANICS OF SINGING

A quotation from Nellie Melba comes to mind. "We would not accept tuition in architecture, chemistry or law from any casual dabbler in these professions, but we welcome the gospel of vocalization from people who have not even a perfunctory acquaintance with the science of singing" (quoted in Weschberg, 1961, p. 212).

Those of us who have chosen teaching as a profession must take time to determine what each student has to work with and how he or she can elicit desired sounds. Nature's way is not only the most healthy, it is also the most beautiful.

While a teacher may not be a professional soloist, just as an athletic coach may not be a champion at his sport, if he has mastered his own voice sufficiently to illustrate what he wants from his students, then he can better empathize with their needs. I pride myself on being able to do with my voice almost anything I ask of my students.

Here is where a knowledge of anatomy and physiology and all other sciences pertaining to voice use can be of value. If you do not know the potential and the limits of the human voice, how can you tell how much or how little to expect from a student?

I repeat what Brodnitz has said many times, that anyone working with the voice needs a well trained and sensitive ear. No matter how much you can see, the ear can tell you things you will never see. I sometimes close my eyes so that I can concentrate better on what I am hearing.

Our beginnings in the "science of singing" date from 1855 when Manual Garcia presented his paper *Observations on the Human Voice* at a meeting of the Royal Society of London. His final writing, *Hints on Singing* dates from 1894. The most complete text for students and teachers of singing since that time has undoubtedly been *Singing, The Mechanism and the Technic* by William Vennard (1967).

Vennard's book is a valuable source of information about the anatomy and physiology of voice as it applies to singers. His chapter on acoustics emphasizes the importance of understanding the physics of sound. While Vennard was working on the scientific aspects of voice, I was working with the clinical applications of those principles. We served together on the Research Committee of the National Association of Teachers of Singing (NATS) and, when he was president of the association, I worked under him as Chairman of the Committee on Vocal Education.

In paragraph 264 of his book, Vennard states in reference to falsetto, "The development of the 'unused register' produces two good results. It builds muscular strength somewhere in the vocal instrument which I shall not venture to identify, but which I am sure is valuable to the singer. Second, this practice gives the singer a 'feel' of something that he should be doing but which he probably does not when he uses only the other mechanism" (p. 76). And again in paragraphs 692 and 693, "The one thing that all must achieve is coordination . . . . The foundation for teaching this is a knowledge of what is being coordinated. There remains a great deal to be discovered by the scientists" (p. 191).

In his book *The Diagnosis and Correction of Vocal Faults*, James McKinney (1982), who studied with Vennard, makes the statement, "There are some who believe that the true upper voice is the falsetto and others who think it is a matter of mixed or blended registers. Until more refined research techniques are available, the determination will rest with the sound which singers produce" (p. 103). And several years later, Sundberg (1987) writes, "However, we are unfortunately still far from a complete understanding of the physiology of register function" (p. 53).

I feel we are getting nearer to the answers to many of these questions. Ingo Titze (1992) points out that "muscles frequently work as agonist-antagonist pairs. The agonist moves a structure in one direction, while the antagonist moves it in the other direction" (p. 21). I have frequently called attention to the contribution of the cricothyroid muscles working against the action of the thyroarytenoids.

In my first year at Barnes Hospital, in 1952, a young man came to me who had studied singing for fifteen years. He had been with four different teachers during that time, all training him as a baritone. On testing his singing, I found he had hardly an octave of usable range, from middle C down one octave. The lower notes were so unsteady that is was difficult to be sure what pitch he was singing. This was a challenge!

I asked the young man to come to my studio where I could work with him more easily. The first time I played A (440 Hz) and asked him to try to sing it, I thought he would faint. He had been told that any falsetto production would ruin his voice. I sang the note myself and asked him to imitate me. After trying it, I asked him if it hurt him in any way. He said no—that he always knew he could make a sound like that but he didn't dare to do so. To make a long story very short, he turned out to be a beautiful lyric tenor. When I last heard of him, he had held the solo position in a large church for over twenty years .

With respect to balancing opposing forces, I have said that if we were to use 100% air with no laryngeal resistance, there would be no sound. Inversely, if we set the laryngeal muscles

100% in resistance, no air could pass through, and again there would be no sound. The ideal for healthy, efficient phonation might be represented by 51% of airflow and 49% glottal resistance. An unrealistic ideal? I'll hold on to it until someone shows me a better way to train the laryngeal mechanism for the demands of musical performance. In my experience it works, so I offer the challenge to other teachers to test it in their "laboratories."

At the beginning of study, both the breathing and the voice are underdeveloped. A coordinated balance of energies is needed so that neither puts undue stress on the other. Breath pressure must be in balance with the condition of the vocal folds. The voice needs time for growth.

CONDUCTING A "MUSICAL HISTORY"

It is important to have as complete a history of your students as possible. A young man came to me for study with so much air passing through his nose that I could hardly understand him, yet a medical examination showed nothing wrong. I was puzzled until he said, "I wonder if my accident had anything to do with this?"

He explained that he had had buck teeth (upper teeth protruding excessively) until he was about 24. At that time, he had been in an accident, and all of his upper teeth were knocked out. His dentures appeared to be normal teeth, so I never guessed that he had learned to talk with this handicap. Imagine what it would be like if you learned to speak without being able to form labial, labiodental, dental, or alveolar consonants and, in addition, had a problem with nasality.

We started on articulation drills, which he followed very well. Finally he exclaimed in his old nasal voice, "Do you mean to say that that's all that's wrong with me?" This question, expressed in his former manner of speaking, sounded hilarious but I couldn't laugh. I only assured him and explained how his nasality had come about.

Know the age of your new students. What is their musical background? Do they have an unusual medical history? What experience have they had singing in choirs and at what age did they start? How long have they studied, and how do they feel about their experiences?

It is not important to know the names of teachers a student has studied with previously. (If the student is from another city, it might be of some value to know who the former teacher was in case you have a student who is moving to that city.) Find out a little about the student's family—how many brothers and sisters, and so on. Also, ask the student about his or her objectives. What kind of music does he or she like best?

I usually ask new students what they think they need—what they feel their problems are. Are there any technical difficulties that they can identify? Singing a song at the first meeting can prove very informative. It will not only show you where students are in their technical development but it will also show what kind of a musician they are. Even more important, it will show you whether they have anything to say in a song.

I remember a soprano with a lovely voice and a good background in music who auditioned at Juilliard. There were no obvious technical difficulties and she had perfect pitch and rhythm. The difficulty was that she left us entirely untouched by what she sang. She might as well have been a mechanical doll reading a laundry list. She was not invited to the school.

Throughout this book, I have called attention to the speaking voice. In an audition, I like to have some conversation with the singer so that I can evaluate whether the speaking pitch seems natural and the phonation and articulation free. Sometimes you can also get a better sense of what kind of field students might thrive in—perhaps something they have not tried—lyric, folk, Broadway.

A bit of vocalizing shows more about voice category and quality. If there are faulty habits carried over from speech and you have not had training in speech therapy yourself, the student should probably see a speech therapist for an evaluation. It is not uncommon to delay singing lessons until speech habits are corrected. A university voice teacher, and former member of the Metropolitan Opera, once brought a student to me for voice therapy. He continued to give her credit for her study, but their lessons were devoted to language, diction, discussions of style, and interpretation. There was no singing until her speaking voice was straightened out.

That teacher was an esteemed colleague and friend who frankly admitted what he could do and what he couldn't. He said to me one time, "If I get a bad student, I'm a bad teacher. If I get a good student, I'm a good teacher." Many of you undoubtedly know of teachers who only accept students with no special problems and therefore have the reputation of being very good. This is important for students to keep in mind in selecting a teacher.

WORKING WITH EXPECTATIONS

I remember a student who came from Washington, D.C., to audition for me. He sang very beautifully, but since he was in financial straits, I advised him to save the money and time it would take him to come to New York and to continue with his teacher in Washington. He became a highly respected professional artist. I lost a student but made a friend.

Young new teachers often expect too much from their students. I sometimes suggest to these teachers how marvelous it would be if a student were able to master just one new idea each lesson.

It is much better to go too slowly than too fast. When students undertake advanced music before their voice is technically ready for it, they will overdo, overreach, and hyperfunction in order to perform the selection. In this regard, I am very much against presenting operatic arias to young students. Many of these pieces were written for fully mature voices, often for a particular artist whom the composer admired. For example, the Prologue to *Pagliaci* was created for Victor Maurel, perhaps the greatest singing actor of his day. When Leoncavallo asked him to create the role of Tonio, Maurel turned him down because there was no aria. So Leoncavallo created the Prologue, which was not a part of the score as first conceived.

A positive approach is very valuable in working with students. I never say "You're doing that wrong." Instead, I suggest, "Let's try another way and see if the voice is ready for it now." If that doesn't work, I admit that it is not going the way we would like and suggest trying a different way. Remember, no two students are alike!

After a short time, I ask students to demonstrate to me how they practice at home. (When students are away from the studio, they are their own teacher.) "Teacher, what are you teaching?" I say. It is amazing to learn what students do on their own. I am often puzzled as to where they get their ideas.

Students often try to hear themselves rather than concentrate on what the singing feels like. That is why I ask students to tell me their sensations, especially if they do not feel comfortable with a tone or scale. Teaching must be a two way process—teacher tells student, student tells teacher.

To help students observe for themselves what is taking place in a lesson, try a tape recorder. I also ask the student to use one of the best teachers they have at home: a mirror. With a mirror and a tape recorder, students can learn to be objective—to observe themselves as though they were monitoring another person.

It is usually desirable to see beginning students for shorter periods of time rather than, say, an hour. Two half-hour lessons or three twenty-minute sessions per week are of much more value early in the learning process. Muscles must be brought into play to carry out tasks they have not been in the habit of performing. These muscles are very small and need time to grow at a natural pace. To quote a saying of Arthur Wilson, "It is better to walk with Mother Nature at your side than ahead of her."

If finances are a problem—and even if they are not—there is great value in having a class of perhaps four students for an hour, especially if they are just starting. Many of the same basic ideas need to be introduced, so instead of saying them four times, you can say them just once. More importantly, it is often easier for a student to identify with what someone else is doing than to be aware of what he or she is doing him- or herself. I have found groups of students to be very supportive of one another. This in itself is tremendously reassuring to each student. In addition, there is a definite feeling of wanting to do one's best among peers.

I have frequently held group lessons with more advanced students as well, both for the sake of the economy and for the opportunity it provides students to get used to singing before others. These classes are very popular. Individuals may take a private lesson in between group lessons. But often I find that students working in groups progress as well as they would in private study.

Repertoire classes are great for advanced students. They offer a valuable way to expand their knowledge of literature and interpretation without having to perform each selection individually. Such classes are often taught by a coach or music historian who can give background information on authors and composers, contextual information frequently neglected by private teachers focusing on technical mastery. For students working toward a performance, both the background and technique are desirable.

When students have special problems, it is much better to have several short lessons each week to help keep him or her on track. Such individual attention does not work well in a group because it is boring to sit and listen while another is struggling. Also the one with the problem is likely to be self-conscious about the difficulty and reluctant to expose his or her weakness in the presence of others.

TEACHING FOR THE LOVE OF IT

I believe most singing teachers love their work. I know that is why I have been at it for so many years. Teaching students one at a time can create strong emotional bonds. A word of caution in this regard: We must realize that students are the product of many influences—often many teachers. I teach to help students learn and grow. If a student feels he or she can learn more in another situation, then I wish him or her the best and hope that it works out that way. I like to feel that anyone who has ever studied with me is always my friend. So far, I have been pretty lucky with this approach.

Some years ago, a young teacher came to my summer seminar from a small midwestern college where she was employed. She told me she hoped she could find a position in a larger school where she would have better students. After returning to her school in the fall, she wrote me a letter in which she stated that she had learned at the seminar that it takes a very broad base to support the career of a great artist and added that she now felt differently about the students she was working with. She was quite content to help each find his potential and learn about the art of singing.

Certainly, everyone who studies voice does not do so with the idea that he or she will be a star. If that were the case, we would have many fewer students and teachers. If a teacher does not empathize with the student's objectives, then the teacher ought not to accept that student.

No teacher should promise success for any student, no matter what the talent. The most a teacher can do is to give an honest opinion about the students' potential and offer to guide them through the hard work it will take to develop their abilities. Certainly a teacher should offer moral support. If students have chosen to study singing out of earnest love of song, they should have a realistic and healthy attitude about their potential.

James King recently said to me, "I think teaching someone to sing is one of the hardest things in the world." I felt like saying, "If you think teaching is hard, you should try writing about it!"

Sometimes I wish I could be young again and study voice with what I know about it today. But, putting sentimental thoughts aside, I know it is because I have struggled to understand my own voice that I can work effectively with my students. If you teach singing, I recommend that you continue to learn all you can about your own voice. We all have a capacity for empathy, but like all virtues, it must be exercised and enlarged.

I sincerely hope that the ideas I have suggested will lead the profession of voice instruction closer to a point where at least no harm is done in the training process. Above all else, it is my hope that what is presented will open the door for as many as possible to learn how to study and develop their voices in a healthy manner.

REFERENCES

Garcia, M. (1894). *Hints on singing*, London: Aschenberg, Hopwood.

McKinney, J. C. (1982). *The diagnosis and correction of vocal faults*, Nashville, Tn: Boardman Press.

Sundberg, J. (1987). *The science of the singing voice*, Decalb, Il: Northern Illinois University Press.

Titze, I. (1992). *Voice quality*, Part I, NATS Journal, May/June, (p. 21).

Vennard, W. (1967). *Singing: the mechanism and the technic*, New York: Carl Fischer.

Wechsberg, J. (1961). *Red plush and black vevet*, Boston: Little, Brown.

BIBLIOGRAPHY

Ackerman, D. (1990). *A natural history of the senses.* New York: Random House.

Adler, K. (1967). *Phonation and diction in singing.* Minneapolis, MN: University of Minnesota Press.

Alderson, R. (1979). *Complete handbook of voice training.* West Nyack, NY: Parker.

Alexander, F. M. (1969). *The resurrection of the body.* New York: University Books.

Andreas, E., & Fowells, R. N. (1970). *The voice of singing.* New York: Carl Fischer.

Anthropology Today. (1971). Communications Research Machine Co. Del Mar, California.

Apel, W. (1965). *Harvard dictionary of music.* Cambridge, MA: Harvard University Press.

Appelman, D. R. (1967). *The science of vocal pedagogy.* Bloomington, IN: Indiana University Press.

Apthorp, W. F. (1901). *The opera past and present.* New York: Scribner's.

Ardoin, J. (1987). *Callas at Julliard.* New York: Knopf.

Arnold, G. E. (1955). Vocal rehabilitation of paralytic dysphonia. *Archives of Otolaryngology, 62*(1).

Bach, A. B. (1884). *Music education and vocal culture.* Edinburgh, Scotland: William Blackwood and Sons.

Bachner, L. (1944). *Dynamic singing.* New York: L. B. Fisher.

Bacon, R. M. (1966). *Elements of vocal science.* Minneapolis, MN: Pro Muscia Press. (Original work published 1824)

Baken, R. J. (1979). Respiratory mechanisms: Introduction and overview. *Transcripts of the 8th Symposium, Care of the professional voice.* New York: The Voice Foundation.

Baken, R. J., & Cavallo, S. A. (1979). Chest wall preparation in the trained speaker. *Transcripts of the 8th Symposium, Care of the professional voice.* New York: The Voice Foundation.

Baken, R. J., & Orlikoff, R. F. (1987). The effect of articulation on fundamental frequency in singers and speakers. *Journal of Voice, 1*(1).

Baker, D. C., Jr. (1962). Laryngeal problems in singers. Transcripts. *American Laryngological Rhinological and Otological Society.*

Baker, G. (1967). *The common sense of singing.* New York: Macmillan.

Balk, H. W. (1979). *The complete singing actor.* Minneapolis, MN: University of Minnesota Press.

Barbeau, P. M. (1941). *Vocal resonance: Its source and command.* New York: Christopher.

Barber, T. X., Spanos, N. P., & Chaves, J. F. (1974). *Hypnosis, imagination and human potentialities.* New York: Pergamon.

Bartholomew, W. T. (1935). The role of imagery in voce *teaching. MTNA Volume of Proceedings.* [reprint]

Bartholomew, W. T. (1942). *Acoustics of music.* New York: Prentice-Hall.

Baryshnikov. (1982, May 16). [Interview] *The New York Times.*

Bechman, G. W. (1955). *Tools for speaking and singing.* New York: Shirmer.

Berard, J. B. (1969). *L'art du chant.* (M. Sidney, Trans.). Minneapolis, MN: Pro Musica Press. (Original work published 1775)

Bernac, P. (1970). *The interpretation of French song.* New York: Norton.

Berry, C. (1973). *Voice and the actor.* New York: Macmillan.

Berry, C. (1981). *Vocal chamber duets: An annotated bibliography.* Jacksonville, FL: National Association of Teachers of Singing.

Berry, M., & Eisenson, J. (1956). *Speech disorders.* New York: Appleton, Century, Crofts.

Bing, R. (1972). *500 nights at the opera.* New York: Popular Library.

Bishop, D. (1991). *The musician as athlete.* Calgary, Canada: Kava.

Bisphan, D. (1920). *A Quaker singer's recollections.* New York: Macmillan.

Black, J. W. (1950). Some effects of auditory stimuli upon voice. *Journal of Aviation Medicine, 22.*

Bless, D. M., & Abbs, J. H. (Eds.). (1983). *Vocal fold physiology.* San Diego, CA: College-Hill Press.

Boland, J. L., Jr. (1953, May). Voice therapy for hoarse voice. *Journal of the Oklahoma State Medical Association, 46.*

Bolles, E. B. (1972, March 18). The innate grammar of baby talk. *Saturday Review.*

Boone, D. R. (1971). *The voice and voice therapy.* New York: Prentice-Hall.

Boone, D. R. (1988). Respiratory training in voice therapy. *Journal of Voice, 2* (#1).

Bordman, G. (1981). *American operetta.* New York: Oxford University Press.

Bouhuys, A., Procter, D. F., & Mead, J. (1966). Kinetic aspects of singing. *Journal of Applied Physiology, 21*(2).

Bradley, B. (1975, April/May). How to approach the changing voice. *The American Music Teacher.*

Brain, J. D., Proctor, D. F., & Reid, L. M. (1977). *Respiratory defense mechanism: Monograph No. 3, Lung biology in health and disease.* New York: Marcel Dekker.

Brandvik, P. (1978). *The complete madrigal dinner book.* Minneapolois, MN: Curtis Music Press.

Briess, F. B. (1957). Voice therapy, Part I. *AMA Archives of Otolaryngology, 66.*

Briess, F. B. (1959). Voice therapy, Part II. *AMA Archives of Otolaryngology, 69.*

Brigance, W. N., & Henderson, F. M. (1945). *A drill manual for improving speech.* Philadelphia: Lippincott.

Brodnitz, F. S. (1953). *Keep your voice healthy.* New York: Harper & Brothers.

Brodnitz, F. S. (1959). *Vocal rehabilitation.* Rochester, MN: Whiting Press.

Brodnitz, F. S. (Chair). (1978). Medical care of the professional voice: Panel discussion. *Transcripts of the 7th Symposium, Care of the professional voice, Part III.* New York: The Voice Foundation.

Brodnitz, F. S. (1979). Psychological consideration in voice therapy. *Transcripts of the 8th Symposium, Care of the professional voice, Part III.* New York: The Voice Foundation.

Brodnitz, F. S., & Froeschels, E. (1954). Treatment of nodules of the vocal cords by the chewing method. *Archives of Otolaryngology, 59.*

Brody, J. E. (1986, June 10). Doctors study treatment of ills brought on by stress. *The New York Times* (C14).

Brody, J. E. (1986, June 11). Safe levels of exercise. *The New York Times.*

Brouillet, G. A. (1916). *Science in vocal production.* Boston: Boston Text Book.

Brown, B. B. (1974). New mind, new body. New York: Harper & Row.

Brown, B. B. (1975, February 22). Biofeedback: An exercise in self-control. *Saturday Review.*

Brown, O. L. (1953, May/June). Principles of voice therapy as applied to teaching. NATS Bulletin.

Brown, O. L. (1958, December). Causes of voice strain in singing. *NATS Bulletin.*

Brown, O. L. (1983). *Voice therapy for singers, I and II.* [video cassettes]. Philadelphia: The Voice Foundation.

Brown, O. L. (1985). Application of research in breathing. *Transcripts of the 14th Symposium, Care of the professional voice.* New York: The Voice Foundation.

Brown, W. E. (1968). *Vocal wisdom: Maxims of Giovanni Battista Lamperti.* New York: Arno Press.

Browne, L., & Benhke, E. (1884). *Voice, song and speech.* New York: Putnam.

Buckley, W. D. (1965). *The solo song cycle: An annotated bibliography.* Ann Arbor, MI: University microfilm.

Buerki, F. A. (1983). *Stagecraft for nonprofessionals.* Madison, WI: University of Wisconsin Press.

Bunch, M. (1982). *Dynamics of the singing voice.* New York: Springer-Verlag.

Burgin, J. (1973). *Teaching singing.* Metuchen, NJ: Scarecrow Press.

Bushnell, H. (1979). *Maria Malibran.* University Park, PA: Pennsylvania State University Press.

Carmen, J. E., et al. (1976). *Art song in the U.S.: An annotated bibliography.* Jacksonville, FL: National Association of Teachers of Singing.

Caruso, D. (1945). *Enrico Caruso.* New York: Simon & Shuster.

Caruso, E. (1973). *How to sing.* Brooklyn, NY: The Opera Box.

Caruso, E., & Tetrazzini, L. (1975). *On the art of singing.* New York: Dover.

Chaliapine, F. (1927). *Pages from my life.* New York: Harper & Row.

Chaliapine, F. (1932). *Man and mask.* Garden City, New York: Doubleday.

Chapman, A. H. (1962). *Management of emotional disorders.* Philadelphia: Lippincott.

Christy, V. A. (1961). *Expressive singing* (vol. I, II). Dubuque, IA: Brown.

Christy, V. A. (1961). *Song anthology* (vol I, II). Dubuque, IA: Brown.

Clippinger, D. A. (1929). *Fundamentals of voice training.* Philadelphia: Oliver Ditson.

Clippinger, D. A. (1932). *The Clippinger class method of voice culture.* Philadelphia: Oliver Ditson.

Coffin, B. (1964). *Phonetic readings of songs and arias.* Boulder, CO: Pruett Press.

Coffin, B. (1976). *The sounds of singing.* Boulder, CO: Pruett Press.

Cogan, R., & Escot, P. (1976). *Sonic Design: The nature of sound and music.* Engelwood Cliffs, NJ: Prentice-Hall.

Cohen, S. J. (1879). *The throat and the voice.* Philadelphia: Lindsay & Blakeston.

Coleman, R. F. (1979). Update on voice registers. *Transcripts of the 8th Symposium, Part I, Care of the professional voice.* New York: The Voice Foundation.

Coleman, R. F. (Chair). (1980). Areas and directions of research in singing. Panel discussion. *Transcripts of the 9th Symposium, Part I, Care of the professional voice.* New York: The Voice Foundation.

Colorni, E. (1976). *Singer's Italian.* New York: Schirmer.

Colton, R. H. (1972). Spectral characteristics of the modal and falsetto registers. *Folia Phoniatrica, 24.*

Colton, R. H. (1988). Physiological mechanisms of vocal frequency control. *Journal of Voice, 2* (3).

Colton, R. H., & Hollein, H. (1973). Perceptual differentiation of the modal and falsetto registers. *Folia Phoniatrica, 25.*

Cone, R. W. (1908). *The speaking voice.* Boston: Evans Music.

Cooksey, J. M. (1977, October). The development of a contemporary. *The Choral Journal.*

Cooper, M. (1973). *Modern techniques of vocal rehabilitation.* Springfield, IL: Charles C. Thomas.

Cooper, M. (1984). *Change your voice, change your life.* New York: Macmillan.

Cox, R. G. (1970). *The singer's Manual of German and French diction.* New York: Schirmer.

Craig, D. (1978). *On singing onstage.* New York: Schirmer.

Craig W. C., & Sokolowskyk, R. B. (1946). *The preacher's voice.* Columbus, OH: Wartburg Press.

Crowest, F. J. (1889). *Advice to singers.* London: Frederick Warne.

Crutchfield, W. (1991, May 24). Homespun virtues still drive a reigning diva. *The New York Times,* Art and Leisure Section.

Culpepper. (1957). Unpublished doctoral dissertation, Nashville, Tn: Peabody College.

Culver, C. A. (1941). *Muscial acoustics.* Philadelphia: Blakiston.

Curtis, H. H. (1973). *Voice building and tone placing* (3rd ed.). Minneappolis, MN: Pro Musica Press. (Original work published 1896)

Curtis, J., Jackobsen, S., & Marcus, E. M. (1972). *An introducation to the neurosciences.* Philadelphia: Sauders.

Daitz, S. (1978). *A recital of ancient greek poetry.* New York: Norton.

Daniell, W. H. (1894). *How to sing.* New York: Fowler & Wells.

Darwin, C. (1968). *The origin of species.* New York: Penguin. (original work published 1859).

Darwin, C. (1896). *The expression of the emotions in man and animals.* New York: Appleton.

Dedo, H. H., & Shipp, T. (1980). *Spastic dysphonia.* Houston, TX: College-Hill Press.

De L'isere, C. (1845). *Diseases and hygiene of the voice.* (J. F. W. Lane, Trans.). Boston: Otis, Borden.

Dorland, W. A. N. (1951). *The American illustrated medical dictionary.* Philadelphia: Saunders.

Douglas, T. E. (1950) Hoarseness. *Northwest Medicine, 49*(6.)

Duey, P. (1951). *Bel canto in its golden age.* New York: King's Crown Press.

Dunbar, F. (1947). *Mind and body: Psychosomatic medicine.* New York: Randon House.

Dunkley, F. (1942). *The buoyant voice.* Boston: Birchard.

Dweyer, E. J. (Ed.) (1972). *Singers in New York.* New York: William Frederick Press.

Eames E. (1927). *Some memories and reflections.* New York: Appleton.

Eaton, Q. (1974). *Opera production I.* New York: Da Capo Press.

Eaton, Q. (1974). *Opera production II.* Minneapolis, MN: University of Minnesota Press.

Eberhardt, C. (1973). *A practical guide for choral rehearsals.* Frankfurt, Germany: Henry Lotolffs Verlag.

Elson, L. C. (1903). *Elson's music dictionary.* Boston: Oliver Ditson.

Emmons, S. (1990). *Tristanissimo.* New York: Schirmer.

Emmons, S., & Sonntag, S. (1979). *The art of song recital.* New York: Schirmer Books.

Erdmann-Chadbourne, N., & Chadbourne, E. (1972). *The art of messa di' voce.* New York: Messa di Voce Foundation.

Espina, M. (1965). *Vocal solos for Protestant services.* New York: Vita d' Arte.

Estill, J. (1980). Observations about quality called "belting." *Transcripts of the 10th Symposium, Care of the professional voice, Part II.* New York: The Voice Foundation.

Estill, J. (1981). An analysis of the spectra of four voice qualities. *Transcripts of the 10th Symposium, Care of the professional voice, Part II.* New York: The Voice Foundation.

Estill, J., & Baer, T., Honda, H., Kiyoshi, H., & Harris, K. S. (1983). An EMG study of supralaryngeal activity in six voice qualities. *Transcripts of the 12th Symposium, Care of the professional voice, Part I.* New York: The Voice Foundation.

Evarts, E. V. (1979, September). Brain mechanisms of movement. *Scientific American.*

Fairbanks, G. (1940). *Voice and articulation drillbook.* New York: Harper & Row.

Fantal, H. (1990, March 18). Listeners pay a high price for loud music. *The New York Times.*

Feldenkrais, M. (1972). *Awareness through movement.* New York: Harper & Row.

Ferrier, W. (1955). *The life of Kathleen Ferrier.* London: Hamish Hamilton.

Fields, V. A. (1947). *Training the singing voice.* New York: King's Crown Press.

Fields, V. A. (1952). *The singer's glossary.* Boston: Boston Music.

Fields, V. A. (1977). *Foundation of the singer's art.* New York: Vantage Press.

Fillebrown, T. (1911). *Resonance in singing and speaking.* Boston: Oliver Ditson.

Finck, H. T. (1909). *Success in music.* New York: Scribner's.

Fink, B. R., & Demarest, R. J. (1978). *Laryngeal biomechanics.* Cambridge, MA: Harvard University Press.

Fischer-Dieskau, D. (1977). *The Fischer-Dieskau book of Lieder.* New York: Knopf.

Fischer-Dieskau, D. (1977). *Schubert songs: A biographical study.* New York: Knopf.

Fisher, H. B. (1970). Objective evaluation of therapy for vocal nodules: A case report. *Journal of Speech and Hearing Disorders, 35*(3).

Flanagan, J. L. (1972, April). The synthesis of speech. *Scientific American.*

Foreman, E. (Ed.). (1968). *The Porpora tradition.* Minneapolis: Pro Musica Press.

Fourcin, A. J. (1974). Laryngographic examination of vocal fold vibration. In B. Wyke (Ed.), *Ventilating and phonatory control system.* London: Oxford University Press.

Fourcin, A. J., & Alberton, E. (1971). First application of a new laryngograph. *Medical and Biological Illustrations, 21.*

Fox, D. R. (1969). Spastic dysphonia: A case presentation. *Journal of Speech and Hearing Disorders, 34*(3).

Frangeon-Davies, D. (1907). *The singing of the future.* New York: John Lane.

Freedman, A. O. (1938). Diseases of the ventricle of Morgagni. *Archives of Otolaryngology, 28.*

Freemantel, F. (1946). *High tones and how to sing them.* New York: Freemantel Voice Institute.

Fried, M. P. (Ed.). (1984). *The otolaryngologic clinics of North America.* (vol. 17, 1). Philadelphia: Saunders.

Frisell, A. (1966). *The soprano voice.* Somerville, MA: Bruce Humphries.

Frisell, A. (1968). *The tenor voice.* Somerville, MA: Bruce Humphries.

Frisell, A. (1972). *The baritone voice.* Boston: Crescendo.

Funk, P. (1982). Stage fright. *Stagebill* (p. 6).

Gallwey, W. T. (1974). *The inner game of tennis.* New York: Random House.

Gallwey, W. T. (1976). *Inner tennis.* New York: Random House.

Ganset, R. (1981). *Singing energy.* New York: Gan-Tone.

Garcia, M. (1982). *Hints on singing.* New York: Patelsen's. (Original work published 1894)

Garden, M., & Biancolli, L. (1951). *Mary Garden's story.* New York: Simon & Schuster.

Gardner, W. (1832). *Music of nature.* Boston: Wilkin, Rice, & Kendall.

Gates, G.A. (1992). Performance anxiety (stage fright): Causes and control. (Unpublished paper quoted with permission.)

Gates, G. A., & Montalbo, P. J. (1987). The effect of low-dose B-blockade on performance anxiety in singers. *Journal of Voice, 1*(1). New York: Raven Press.

Gatz, A. J. (1970). *Manter's essentials of clinical neuroanatomy and neurophysiology.* Philadelphia: Davis.

Gelb, M. (1981). *Body learning: An introduction to the Alexander technique.* New York: Delilah Books.

Geshwind, N. (1979, September). Specialization of the human brain. *Scientific American.*

Gibran, K. (1926). *The prophet.* New York: Knopf.

Gilliland, D. V. (1970). *Guildance in vocal education.* Columbus, OH: Typographic Printing.

Glackens, Ira (1963). *Yankee diva.* New York: Coleridge Press.

Glasser, W. (1965). *Reality therapy.* New York: Harper & Row.

Goldowsky, B. (1968). *Bringing opera to life.* New York: Appleton, Century, Crofts.

Gollobin, L. B., & White, H. (1977–1978, December, February, April). Voice teachers on voice. Parts I, II, III. *Music Educator's Journal.*

Gorky, M. (1967). *Chaliapin: An autobiography.* New York: Stein and Day.

Gould W. J. (1971). Effect of respiratory and postural mechanisms upon the action of the vocal folds. *Folia Phoniatrica, 23.*

Gould, W. J. (1979). Interrelationship between voice and laryngeal mucosal reflexes. *Transcripts of the 8th Symposium, Care of the professional voice, Part II.* New York: The Voice Foundation.

Gould, W. J. (1981). The pulmonary-laryngeal system. *Vocal fold physiology.* Tokyo: University of Tokyo Press.

Gould, W. J., & Okamura, H. (1973, January/February). Static lung volumes in singers. *Annals of Otology, Rhinology and Laryngology, 82*(1).

Gould, W. J., & Okamura, H. (1974). Respiratory training of the singer. *Folia Phoniatrica, 26,* 275–286

Gould, W. J., Rubin, J., Korovin, G., & Sataloff, R. T. (1995). *Diagnosis and treatment of voice disorders.* New York: Igaku Shoin.

Gould, W. J., Sataloff, R. T., & Spiegel, J. R. (1973). *Voice surgery.* St. Louis, MO: Mosby.

Graham, M. (1991). *Blood memory.* New York: Washington Square Press.

Gray, G., & Wise, C. (1946). *The bases of speech.* New York: Harper.

Gray, G. W., & Braden, W. W. (1951). *Public speaking.* New York: Harper.

Gray, H. (1954). *Anatomy of the human body* (26th ed.). (C. M. Goss, Ed.). Philadelphia: Lea & Febiger.

Green, B., with Gallwey, W. T. (1986). The inner game of music. New York: Doubleday.

Greene, A. (1975). *The new voice.* New York: Chappel Music.

Greene, M. (1964). *The voice and its disorders.* London: Pitman Medical.

Greenspan, E. (1983, August 28). Conditioning athletic minds. *The New York Times.*

Grubb, T. (1979). *Singing in French.* New York: Schirmer Books.

Guilbert, Y. (1918). *How to sing.* New York: Macmillan.

Guthrie, D. (1939). Discussion of functional disorders of the voice. *Journal of Laryngology and Otolaryngology, 54.*

Harper, R. M. (1940). *The voice governor.* Boston: Schirmer Music.

Harris, T. A. (1969). I'm OK You're OK. New York: Harper & Row.

Hast, M. H. (1983). Comparative anatomy of the larynx: Evolution and function. In I. R. Titze & R. C. Scherer (Eds.). *Vocal fold physiology.* Denver, CO: The Denver Center for the Performing Arts.

Haugen, G. B., et al. (1958). *A therapy for anxiety tension reactions.* New York: Macmillan.

Haywood, F. H. (1948, 1949, 1957). *Universal song* (vols. I, II, III). New York: Schirmer.

Heaton, W., & Hargens, C. W. (1968). *An interdisciplinary index of studies in physics, medicine and music related to the human voice.* Bryn Mawr, PA: Theodore Presser.

Heaver, L. (1962, October). Psychosemantic aspects of nonverbal communications. *Logos, 5* (2).

Heinrich, M. (1910). *Correct priniciples of classical singing.* Boston: Lothrop, Lea & Shephard.

Henahan, D. (1988, March 6). Why singers don't set records. *The New York Times.*

Herbert, C. E. (1958). *Tradition and Gigli.* London: Robert Hale.

Herbert, C. E. (1965). *The alchemy of voice.* London: Robert Hale.

Herbert, C. E. (1969). *Vocal truth.* Boston: Crescendo.

Herbert, C. E. (1971). *The science of sensations of vocal tones.* Boston: Crescendo.

Herbert, C. E. (1971). *The voice of the mind.* London: Robert Hale.

Herrigel, E. (1969). *Zen and the art of archery*. New York: Vintage Books.

Highet, G. (1950). *The art of teaching*. New York: Vintage Books.

Hinchcliffe, R., & Harrison, D. (Eds.). (1976). *Scientific foundations of oto-laryngology*. Chicago: William Heinemann Medical Books.

Hines, J. (1982). *Great singers on great singing*. Garden City, New York: Doubleday.

Hirano, M. (1988). Behavior of laryngeal muscles of the late William Vennard. *Journal of Voice, 2*(4). New York: Raven Press.

Hirano, M. (1988). Vocal mechnaisms in singing: Larynogolgoycal and phoniatric aspects. *Journal of Voice, 2*(1). New York: Raven Press.

Hirano, M., Kiyokawa, K., & Kurita, S. (1988). Laryngeal muscles and glottic shaping. In O. Fujimura (Ed.), *Vocal fold physiology*. New York: Raven Press.

Hirose, H. (1979). Laryngeal EMG. *International Symposium on the Larynx*. San Francisco.

Hirose, H., & Gay, T. (1973). Laryngeal control in vocal attacks. *Folia Phoniatrica, 25*.

Hirsh, I. J. (1952). *The measurement of hearing*. New York: McGraw-Hill.

Hixon, T. J., & Hoffmant, C. (1978). Chest wall shape in singing. *Transcripts of the 7th Symposium, Care of the professional voice, Part I*. New York: The Voice Foundation.

Hixon, T. J., Watson, P. J., Harris, F. P., & Pearl, N. B. (1988). Related volume changes in the rib cage and abdomen during prephonatory chest wall posturing. *Journal of Voice, 2*(1).

Holland, B. (1984, February 19). It takes more than talent to build a musical career. *The New York Times*, Art and Leisure Section (p. 1).

Hollein, H. (1978). The sound and its origin. Panel discussion. *Transcripts of the 7th Symposium, Care of the professional voice, Part I*. New York: The Voice Foundation.

Hollein, H. (1983). A report on vocal registers. *Transcripts of the 12th Symposium, Care of the professional voice, Part I*. New York: The Voice Foundation.

Hollein, H., & Brown, W. S., Jr., & Hollein, K. (1971). Vocal fold length associated with modal, falsetto and varying intensity phonations. *Folia Phoniatrica, 33*.

Hooper, J., and Teresi, D. (1986). *The three pound universe*. New York: Dell.

Hubel, D. H. (1979, September). The brain. *Scientific American*.

Hume, P. (1972). Why do young voices burn out? *Globe-Democrat-Washington Post* News Service.

Husler, F., & Rodd-Marling, Y. (1965). *Singing: The physical nature of the vocal organs*. New York: October House.

Hutchison, M. (1986). *Megabrain*. New York: Beech Tree.

Ingram, M., & Rice, W. (1962). *Vocal technique for children and youth*. New York: Abington Press.

Iverson, L. L. (1979, September). The chemistry of the brain. *Scientific American*.

Jackson, C. (1940, September). Myasthenia laryngis. *Archives of Otolaryngology, 32.*

Jackson, C., & Jackson, C. L. (1937). *The larynx and its diseases.* Philadelphia: Saunders.

Jacobs, A. (1958). *A new dictionary of music.* Baltimore: Penguin.

Jacobson, E. (1952). *Progressive relaxation.* Chicago: University of Chicago Press.

Jacobson, E. (1964). *Anxiety tension control.* Philadelphia: Lippincott.

Janow, A. (1991). *The new primal scream.* Wilmington, DE: Enterprise.

Joiner, J. R. (1988, December). The relationship of the vocal folds to vowel formation: A study of current research. *Journal of Research in Singing, 12*(1).

Jones, F. P. (1976). *Body awareness in action: A study of the Alexander technique.* New York: Schoken Books.

Jones, A. N., Smith, M. I., & Wall, R. B. (1945). *Pronouncing guide to French, German and Spanish.* New York: Carl Fischer.

Journal of Voice. (1987-Present). Journal of the Voice Foundation. New York.

Judson, L. S. V., Lyman, S. V., & Weaver, A. T. (1965). *Voice science.* New York: Appleton-Century-Crofts.

Kagen, S. (1950). *On studying singing.* New York: Dover.

Kagen, S. (1968). *Music for the voice.* Bloomington, IN: Indiana University Press.

Karr, H. (1953). *Developing your speaking voice.* New York: Harper & Row.

Kellog, C. L. (1913). *Memories of an Amerian prima donna.* New York: Putnam's.

Kirchner, J. A. (1983). Factors influencing glottal aperture. In D. M. Bless, & J. H. Abbs (Eds.), *Vocal fold physiology.* San Diego, CA: College-Hill Press.

Kirchner, J. A. (1986). *Vocal fold histopathology.* San Diego, CA: College-Hill Press.

Kirchner, J. A. (1988). *Fundamental evolution of the human larynx: Variations among the vertebrates.* New York: Raven Press.

Kirsten, D. (1975, December 30). From group interview. *The New York Times.*

Kitzing, P., & Soneson, B. (1967). Shape and shift of the laryngeal ventrical during phonation. *Acta Oto-laryngologica, 63.*

Klausoto, H. A. (1986). *Writing on both sides of the brain.* New York: Harper & Row.

Klein, H. (1920). *The Reign of Patti.* New York: The Century Co.

Klein, J. (1967). *Singing techniques.* Princeton, NJ: Van Nostrand.

Kofler, L. (1887). *The art of breathing.* New York: Edgar S. Werner.

Koyama, T., Kawasaki, M., & Ogura, J. (1969). Mechanics of voice production, I: Regulation of vocal intensity. *The Laryngoscope, LXXIX*(3).

Kraines, S. H. (1948). *The therapy of the neuroses and psychoses.* Philadelphia: Lea & Febiger.

Kurtz, R., & Prestera, H. (1976). *The body reveals.* New York: Harper & Row.

La Barre, W. (1954). *The human animal.* Chicago: The University of Chicago Press.

Ladefoged, P. (1962). *Elements of acoustic phonetics.* Chicago: The University of Chicago Press.

Lamperti, F. (18—). *A treatise on the art of singing.* (J. C. Griffith, Trans.). New York: Edward Schuberth.

Lang, P. H. (1971). *Critic at the opera.* New York: Norton.

Large, J. (1980). *Contributions of voice research to singing* Houston, TX: College-Hill Press.

Large, J., & Iwata, S. (1971). Aerodynamic study of vibrato and voluntary 'straight tone' pairs in singing. *Folia Phoniatrica, 23.*

Larson, C. R. (1988). Brain mechanisms involved in the control of vocalization. *Journal of Voice, 2*(4). New York: Raven Press.

Lawrence, M. (1949). *Interrupted melody.* New York: Appleton-Century-Crofts.

Lawrence, V. L. (Ed.). (1977, June–1985, June). *Transcripts of the Symposium, Care of the professional voice.* New York: The Voice Foundation.

Lawton, M. (1929). *Schumann-Heink.* New York: Macmillan.

Leanderson, R. (1972). On the functional organization of the facial muscles in speech. *Acta Otolaryngology.*

Leanderson, R., Sundberg, J., von Euler, C., & Lagercrantz, H. (1983). Diaphragmatic control of the subglottic pressure during singing. *Transcripts of the 12th Symposium, Care of the professional voice.* New York: The Voice Foundation.

Leanderson, R., Sundberg, J., & von Euler, C. (1984). Effects of diaphragm activity during singing. *Transcripts of the 12th Symposium, Care of the professional voice.* New York: The Voice Foundation.

Leanderson, R., Sundberg, J., & von Euler, C. (1987). Role of diaphragmatic activity during singing. *Journal of Applied Physiology, 62.*

Leanderson, R., & Sunberg, J. (1988). Breathing for singing. *Journal of Voice, 2*(1).

Lehmann, L. (1909). *How to sing.* (R. Aldrich, Trans.). New York: Macmillan.

Lehmann, L. (1938). *Midway in my song.* Indianapolis, IN: Bobbs-Merrill.

Lehmann, L. (1971). *Eighteen song cycles.* London: Cassel.

Leonard, G. (1975, February 22). In God's image. *Saturday Review.*

Lessac, A. (1973). *The use and training of the human voice.* New York: Drama Book.

LeVan, T. (1991). *Masters of the French art song.* New York: Scarecrow Press.

Lewis, R. (1980). *Advice to the players.* New York: Harper & Row.

Leyerle, W. (1977). *Vocal development through organic imagery.* New York: State University of New York Press.

Liberman, P. (1988, July/August). Voice in the wilderness. *The Sciences.*

L'Isere, C. de (1845). *Treatise upon the diseases and hygiene of the organs of the voice* (J. F. W. Lane, Trans.). Boston: Otis, Broaders.

Lloyd, L., & deGaetani, J. (1980). *The complete sightsinger.* New York: Harper & Row.

Logos: The Bulletin of the National Hospital for Speech Disorders (1958–1963). Vols 1–6. New York.

Lowen, A. (1972). *Depression and the body.* London: Penguin.

Lowen, A. (1975). *Bioenergetics.* New York: Penguin.

Lowen, A. (1979). *The language of the body.* New York: Collier.

Lucksinger, R., & Arnold, G. (1965). *Voice speech language.* Belmont, CA: Wordsworth.

MacClintock, C. (1973). *The solo song: 1580–1730.* New York: Norton.

MacCurtain, F., Metz, D. E., Reed, V. W. (1981). Measurement of voice quality at the source. Panel discussion. *Transcripts of the 10th Symposium, Care of the professional voice, Part II.* New York: The Voice Foundation.

Mackenzie, M. (1891). *The hygiene of the vocal organs.* New York: Werner.

Maltz, M. (1972). *Psycho-Cybernetics.* New York: Pocket Books.

Mancini, G. (1967). *Practical reflections on figured singing.* E. Foreman (Ed.). Minneapolis, MN: Pro Musica Press. (Original publication 1774).

Manen, L. (1974). *The art of singing.* London: Faber Music.

Marafioti, P. M. (1981). *Caruso's method of voice production.* New York: Dover. (Original work published 1922)

Marchesi, M. (1901). *Ten singing lessons.* New York: Harper.

Marshall, M. (1966). *The singer's manual of English diction.* New York: Schirmer.

Masters, R. (1975, February, 22). The psychophysical experience. *Saturday Review.*

May, R. (1975). *The courage to create.* New York: Bantam.

McArthur, E. (1965). *Flagstad.* New York: Knopf.

McCall, G. (1977). Projected research concerned with central neurological pathologies on laryngeal dysfunction. *Transcripts of the 6th Symposium, Care of the professional voice.* New York: The Voice Foundation.

McCloskey, D. B. (1969). *Your voice at its best.* Boston: Little, Brown.

McCloskey, D. B., & Barbara, H. (1975). *Voice in song and speech.* Boston: Boston Music.

McCormack, J. (1918). *John McCormack: His own life story.* Boston: Small, Maynard.

McKinney, J. C. (1982). *The diagnosis and corrections of vocal faults.* Nashville, TN: Broadman Press.

McLellan, E. (1920). *Voice education.* New York: Harper.

Mead, M. (1970). *Culture and commitment.* Garden City, New York: Doubleday.

Meador, C. L., & Myskens, A. (1950). *Handbook of biolinguistics, Part I.* Toledo, OH: Weller.

Meador, C. L., & Myskens, A. (1959). *Handbook of biolinguistics: General semantics.* Toledo, OH: Weller.

Meano, C., & Khoury, A. (1967). *The human voice in speech and song.* Springfield, IL: Charles C. Thomas.

Memory. (1986, September 29). Article in *Newsweek.*

Miller, F. (1910). *Vocal art science.* New York: Schirmer.

Miller, F. (1917). *The voice.* New York: Schirmer.

Miller, L. (1983, June 6). Stress: Can we cope? *Time*.

Miller, P. (1966). *The ring of words*. Garden City, New York: Doubleday.

Miller, R. (1977). *Techniques of singing*. Metuchen, NJ: Scarecrow Press.

Miller, R. (1986). *The structure of singing*. New York: Schirmer Books.

Miller, R., & Schutte, H. K. (1981, January/February). The effect of tongue position on spectra in singing. *NATS Bulletin*.

Mills, W. (1908). *Voice production in singing and speaking*. Philadelphia: Lippincott.

Merriam-Webster. (1981). *Eighth new collegiate dictionary*. Springfield, MA: Merriam-Webster.

Monahan, B. J. (1978). *The art of singing: A compendium of thoughts on singing published between 1777 and 1927*. Metuchen, NJ: Scarecrow Press.

Moore, G. P. (1971). *Organic voice disorders*. Englewood Cliffs, NJ: Prentice-Hall.

Moriarity, J. (1975). *Diction: Italian, Latin, French, German*. Boston: Schirmer Music.

Moses, P. J. (1954). *The voice of neurosis*. New York: Grune & Stratton.

Mott, F. W. (1910). *The brain and the voice in speech and song*. New York: Harper.

Meyer, E. J. (1902). *The renaissance of the vocal art*. Boston: Boston Music.

Myerson, M. C. (1955, June). Observations and considerations on cigarette smoking. *Annals of Otology, Rhinology and Laryngology, 2*.

NATS Bulletin. (1992, November/December). The role of the speech-language pathologist and teacher of singing in remediation of singers with voice disorders (p. 14).

Nauta, W. J. H., & Freitag, M. (1979, September). The organization of the brain. *Scientific American*.

Negus, V. E. (1938, September). Evolution of the speech organs of man. *Archives of Otolaryngology, 28*.

Neubauer, E. J. (1937, September). Turning the falsetto to account. *The Etude*.

Newson, F. (1968). *Guide for young singers*. New York: William Frederick Press.

Newton, G. (1984). *Sonority in singing*. New York: Vantage Press.

Nicoll, I. H. (1940). *Simplified vocal training*. New York: Carl Fischer.

Nilsson, L., & Lindberg, J. (1974). *Behold man*. (A. B. Folag, Trans.). Boston: Little, Brown.

Nordica, L. (1923). *Hints to singers*. (W. Armstrong, Editor). New York: Dutton.

Orrey, L. (Ed.). (1976). *The encyclopedia of opera*. New York: Scribner's.

Osborne, C. L. (1979, January). The Broadway voice. *High Fidelity*.

Ostwald, P. F. (1963). *Soundmaking*. Springfield, IL: Charles C. Thomas.

Owens, R. (1983). *Towards a career in Europe*. Dallas, TX: AMS.

Owens, R. (1984). *The professional singer's guide*. Dallas, TX: AMS.

Panzera, C. (1964). *Melodies Francais*. New York: C. F. Peters.

Paschke, D. V. (Ed. and Trans.). (1975). *Manuel Garcia II: A complete treatise on the art of singing, Part II* (1847 and 1872 eds.). New York: Da Capo Press.

Pattou, A. A. (1878). *The voice as an instrument.* [typed copy]. The Julliard Library, New York.

Peck, M. S. (1978). *The road less traveled.* New York: Touchstone.

Peirce, J. W. (1951). *The art of program making.* Boston: E. C. Schirmer.

Peterson, P. W. (1965). *Criteria for the evaluation of vocal performance.* New York: Brodt Music.

Peterson, W. B., & Kopitzke, C. B. (1976). *Handbook on singing.* Milwaukee, WI: Kard.

Pleasants, H. (1966). *The great singers.* New York: Simon & Shuster.

Powers, M. (1976). *Self hypsosis: Its theory, technique and application.* North Hollywood, CA: Wilshire.

Prawer, S. S. (1964). *The Penguin book of Lieder.* Baltimore: Penguin.

Pressman, J. J. (1940). Physiology of the larynx: A resume and discussion of the literature for 1939. *Laryngoscope, 59*(4).

Pressman, J. J. (1942, March). Physiology of the vocal cords in phonation and respiration. *Archives of Otolaryngology, 35*(3).

Pressman, J. J., & Keleman, G. (1955). *Physiology of the Larynx.* Reprint from Physiological Review, 35(3): American Academy of Ophthamology and Otolaryngology.

Proctor, D. F. (1979). Breath, the power source for the voice. *Transcripts of the 8th Symposium, Care of the professional voice, Part II.* New York: The Voice Foundation.

Proschowsky, F. (1923). *The way to sing.* Boston: Birchard.

Punt, N. A. (1979). *The singer's and actor's throat.* London: Heinemann.

Punt, N. A. (1983). Laryngology applied to singers and actors. *Journal of Laryngology and Otology, 6* (suppl).

Puritz, E. (1956). *The teaching of Elizabeth Schumann.* London: Methuen.

Putman's contemporary Italian dictionary. (1974). New York: Berkley.

Quiring, D. P., & Warfel, J. H. (1960). *The head, neck and trunk.* Philadelphia: Lea & Febiger.

Ray, B. (1985). *The Reiki factor.* St. Petersburg, FL: Radiance Assoc.

Rebner, W., & Bettag, I. (1972). *Approach to new music.* New York: Peters.

Reed, V. W. (1981). *The electroglottograph in voice teaching. Transcripts of the 10th Symposium, Care of the professional voice, Part II.* New York: The Voice Foundation.

Reid, C. L. (1965). *The free voice.* New York: Patelson's Music House.

Reid, C. L. (1972). *Bel canto.* New York: Patelson's Music House.

Reid, C. L. (1975). *Voice: Psyche and soma.* New York: Patelson's Music House.

Restak, R. W. (1984). *The brain.* New York: Bantam.

Ristad, E. (1982). *A soprano on her head.* Moab, UT: Real People Press.

Rose, A. (1962). *The singer and the voice.* London: Faber & Faber.

Resewald, R. B. (1961). *Hanbook of singing.* Evanston, IL: Summy Birchard.

Ross, W. E. (1948). *Sing high, sing low.* New York: Carl Fischer.

Ross, W. E. (1959). *Secrets of singing.* Bloomington, IN: Indiana University Presss.

Rushmore, R. (1971). *The singing voice.* New York: Dodd, Mead.

Russell, F. (1979). *The subject of singing.* Los Alamitos, CA: Hwong.

Sadie, S. (Ed.). (1988). *Norton/Grove concise encyclopedia of music.* New York: Norton.

Sataloff, R. T. (1981). Professional singers: The science and art of clinical care. *American Journal of Otolaryngology, 2*(3).

Sataloff, R. T. (1991). *Professional voice: The science and art of clinical care. New York: Raven Press.*

Sataloff, R. T. (1992). The human voice. *Scientific American, 267* (6), 108-115.

Sataloff, R. T., & Titze, I. R. (Eds.). (1991). *Vocal health and science.* Jacksonville, FL: National Association of Teachers of Singing.

Saunders, W. H. (1956). Dysphonia plica ventricularis. *Annals of Otology, Rhinology and Laryngology, 65*(3).

Saunders, W. H. (1964). *The larynx.* Summit, NJ: CIBA Pharmaceutical Co.

Schiotz, A. (1970). *The singer and his art.* New York: Harper & Row.

Schmidt, J. (1984). *Basics of singing.* New York: Schirmer Books.

Scholes, P. A. (1943). *The Oxford companion of music.* London: Oxford University Press.

Schonberg, H. C. (1981). *Facing the music.* New York: Summit Books.

Schubert, E. D. (1982). On hearing your own performance. *Transcripts of the 11th Symposium, Care of the professional voice, Part I.* New York: The Voice Foundation.

Sendax, V. I. (1981). A dento-facial perspective to the care of the professional voice. *Transcripts of the 10th Symposium, Care of the professional voice, Part II.* New York: The Voice Foundation.

Shakespeare, W. (1910). *The art of singing.* Boston: Oliver Ditson.

Shaw, H. (1980, April). It takes more than virtuosity to build a career. *Fugue* (p. 54).

Sherrington, C. (1947). *The integrative action of the nervous system.* New Haven, CT: Yale University Press.

Shin, T., Hirano, M., Maeyama, T., Nozoe, I., & Ohkubo, H. (1981). The function of the extrinsic laryngeal muscles. In K. N. Stevens & M. Hirano (Eds.), *Vocal fold physiology.* Tokyo: University of Tokyo Press.

Shipp, T. (Chair), Guinn, L., Sundberg, J., and Titze, I. R. (1987). Verticle laryngeal position. [discussion]. *Journal of Voice, 1* (3).

Shultz, G. D. (1962). *Jenny Lind.* Philadelphia: Lippencott.

Sieber, F. (1872). *Art of singing.* (F. Seeger, Trans.). New York: William Pond.

Simonton, O. C. (1978). *Getting well again.* Los Angeles: Tarcher.

Singher, M. (1985). *An interpretive guide to operatic arias.* University Park, PA: Pennsylvania Press.

Slezak, W. (1962). *What time's the next swan?* Garden City, NY: Doubleday.

Smith, K. J. (1981). *The informed performer's dictionary of instruction for the performing arts.* New York: TIP.

Smolover, R. (1971). *The vocal essence.* Scarsdale, NY: Covenant.

Sonninen, A. A. (1956). The role of the external laryngeal muscles in length-adjustment of the vocal cords in singing. *Acta Oto Laryngologica.*

Sonninen, A., & Damste, P. H. (1971). An instructional terminology in the field of logopedics and phoniatrics. *Folia Phoniatrica, 23.*

Sonninen, A., Damste, P. H., Jol, J., Fokkens, J., & Reolofs, J. (1974). Microdynamics in vocal fold vibration. *Acta Otolaryngology, 78.*

Southern, E. (1971). *The music of Black Americans.* New York: Norton.

Speads, C. H. (1978). *Breathing, the ABC's.* New York: Harper & Row.

Stamford, W. B. (1967). *The sound of Greek.* Berkeley, CA: Univeristy of California Press.

Stanislavski, C. (1972). *An actor prepares.* New York: Theatre Art Books.

Stanislavski, C. (1974). *Stanislavski on opera.* New York: Theatre Art Books.

Stanley, D. (1948). *The science of voice.* New York: Carl Fischer.

Starr, D. (1984, June). A window on the brain. *Reader's Digest.*

Sternberg, R. J. (1985). *Human abilities.* New York: Freeman.

Stock, G. C. (1912). *Guiding thoughts for singers.* New Haven, CT: Harty-Musch.

Stockhausen, J. (1884). *Methods of singing.* New York: Novello.

Stoer, V. L., & Swank, H. (1978, December). Mending misused voices. *Music Education Journal.*

Strong, M. S., & Vaughan, C. W. (1981). The morphology of the phonatory organs and their neural control. In K. N. Stevens & M. Hirano (Eds.), *Vocal fold physiology.* Tokyo: University of Tokyo Press.

Sundberg, J. (1974). Acoustic interpretation of the singer's formant. *Journal of the Acoustical Society of America, 55,* 838–844.

Sundberg, J. (1977, March). The acoustics of the singing voice. *Scientific American.*

Sundberg, J. (1987). *The science of the singing voice.* Dekalb, IL: Northern Illinois University Presss.

Swanson, F. J. (1973). *Music teaching in the junior high and middle school.* New York: Appleton, Century, Croft.

Swanson, F. J. (1977). *The male singing voice ages 8–18.* Cedar Rapids, IA: Lawrence Press.

Swanson, F. J. (1977, January). The vanishing basso profundo and fry tones. *The Choral Journal.*

Swisher, W. S. (1927). *Music in worship.* Boston: Oliver Ditson.

Swisher, W. S. (1927). *Psychology for the music teacher.* Boston: Oliver Ditson.

Tate, G. P. (1978). *Functional voice.* Pittsburgh, PA: Volkwein Bros.

Taylor, R. N. (1958). *Acoustics for the singer.* Emporia, KS: Kansas State Teachers College.

Thomas, L. (1975). *The lives of a cell.* Toronto, Canada: Bantam Books.

Thompson, O. (1939). *International cyclopedia of music and musicians.* New York: Dodd, Mead.

Titze, I. R. (1981, May/June). Is there scientific explanation for tone focus and voice placement? *NATS Bulletin.*

Titze, I. R. (1988). A framework for the study of vocal registers. *Journal of Voice, 2*(3).

Titze, I. R. (1988). Regulation of vocal power and efficiency by subglottal pressure and glottal width. In O. Fujimura (Ed.), *Vocal fold physiology.* New York: Raven Press.

Titze, I. R. (1992, May/June). Voice quality, Part I. *NATS Bulletin.*

Titze, I. R. (1994). *Principles of voice production.* Englewood Cliffs, NJ: Prentice-Hall.

Todd, M. E. (1968). *The thinking body.* New York: Dance Horizons.

Togawa, K., & Ogura, J. H. (1966, January). Physiologic relationships between nasal breathing and pulmonary function. *The Laryngoscope, 76.*

Tokay, E. (1944). *Fundamentals of physiology.* New York: Barnes & Noble.

Tosi, P. (1986). *Opinions of singers ancient, and modern, or, observations on figured singing.* (E. Foreman, Trans.). Minneapolis, MN: Pro Musica Press. (Original work published 1723)

Trussler, I., & Ehret, W. (1960). *Functional lessons in singing.* Englewood Cliffs, NJ: Prentice-Hall.

Tubbs, F. H. (1897). *Seed thoughts for singers.* New York: Frank H. Tubbs.

Ulrich, B. (1910). *Concerning the principles of voice training during the a cappella period and the beginning of opera* (1474-1640. (W. Seale, Trans., E. Foreman, Ed.). Minneapolis, MN: Pro Musica Press.

Update on vocal registers. Panel discussion. (1979). *Transcripts of the 8th Symposium, Care of the professional voice, Part I.* New York: The Voice Foundation.

Uris, D. (1971). *To sing in English.* New York: Boosey and Hawkes.

Vaitukaitis, J., & Ross, R. N. (1984, September/October). Hormones. *Bostonia, 58* (6). (Boston University)

Vale, W. S., & Nicholson, S. H. (1932). *The training of boy's voices.* London: Faith Press.

Van Alyea, O. E. (1949). *The embryology of the ear, nose and throat.* Monograph of the American Academy of Ophthamology and Otolaryngology. Omaha, NB: Douglas Printing.

Van Deinse, J. B. (1981). Registers. *Folia Phoniatrica, 33.*

Van Deinse, J. B., & Frateur, L. (1973). *Some remarks on the function of the cricothyroid muscle.* Basel, Switzerland: Separatum.

Van Deinse, J. B. et al. (1974). Problems of the singing voice. *Folia Phoniatrica, 26.*

Van denBerg, J. (1957). On the air resistance and the Bernoulli effect of the human larynx. *Journal of the Aoustical Society of America, 29.*

Van denBerg, J. (1958). Myoelastic-aerodynamic theory of voice production. *Journal of Speech and Hearing Research.*

Van denBerg, J., & Tan, T. S. (1959, November). Results of experiments with human larynxes. *Practica Oto-Rhino-Laryngolica, 21*(6).

Van Riper, C. (1965). *Speech correction.* Englewood Cliffs, NJ: Prentice-Hall.

Vennard, W. (1967). *Singing: The mechanism and the technic.* New York: Carl Fischer.

Vennard, W. (1973). *Developing voices*. New York: Carl Fischer.

Vishnevskaya, G. (1984). *Galina*. San Diego, CA: Harcourt Brace.

Voice quality in the professional world. (1982). Panel discussion. *Transcripts of the 11th Symposium, Care of the professional voice, Part II*. New York: The Voice Foundation.

Von Leden, H. (1982). The cultural history of the human voice. *Transcripts of the 11th Symposium, Care of the professional voice, Part II*. New York: The Voice Foundation.

Walker, J. S. (1988). An investigation of the whistle register in the female voice. *Journal of Voice, 2* (2).

Wall, J., & Weatherspoon, R. (1978). *Anyone can sing*. Garden City, NY: Doubleday.

Wang, S. (1983). Bright timbre, acoustic features and larynx position. Paper presented at the 105th meeting of the Accoustical Society of America, Stockholm, Sweden.

Waters, C. (1930). *Song, the substance of vocal study*. New York: Schirmer.

Watson, P., & Hixon, T. (1985, March). Respiratory kinematics in classical opera singers. *Journal of Speech and Hearing Research, 28*.

Wechsberg, J. (1961). *Red plush and black velvet*. Boston: Little, Brown.

Wedin, S. (1970). E.M.G. investigation of abdominal musculature during phonation. [pamphlet]. Boden, Sweden.

Weinberg, B. (Ed.). (1978). Life-span changes in the human voice. Panel discussion. *Transcripts of the 7th Symposium, Care of the professional voice, Part II*. New York: The Voice Foundation.

Weiss, D. H., & Beebe, H. (1951). *The chewing approach to speech and voice therapy*. New York: Karger.

West, A., Ansberry, M., & Carr, A. (1957). *The rehabilitation of speech*. New York: Harper & Row.

Westerman, K. N. (1955). *The emergent voice*. Ann Arbor, MI: Edwards Bros.

White, E. G. (1950). *Science and singing*. Boston: Crescendo.

White, J. W. (1975, February 22). The consciousness revolution. *Saturday Review*.

Whitlock, W. (1967). *Master lessons on fifty opera arias* (vols. 1, 2). Minneapolis, MN: Pro Musica Press.

Whitlock, W. (1967). *Facets of the singer's art*. Minneapolis, MN: Pro Musica Press.

Wilcox, J. C. (1935). *The living voice*. New York: Carl Fischer.

Wilder, C. N. (1979). Chest wall preparation for phonation in trained speakers. *Transcripts of the 8th Symposium, Care of the professional voice, Part II*. New York: The Voice Foundation.

Wilson, D. K. (1966, November). Voice re-education in benign laryngeal pathology. *The Eye, Ear, Nose and Throat Monthly, 45*.

Winckel, F. (1971). How to measure the effectiveness of stage singer's voices. *Folia Phoniatrica, 23*.

Winsel, R. (1966). *The anatomy of voice*. New York: Exposition Press.

Withrow, M. (1915). *Some staccato notes for singers*. Boston: Oliver Ditson.

Wollitz, K. (1977). The countertenor voice defined. [interview with Jeffrey Dooley]. *The American Recorder*, New York.

Wyke, B. (1974). *Ventilatory and phonatory control systems: International symposium.* London: Oxford University Press.

Wyke, B. (1979). Neurological aspects of phonatory control systems in the larynx. A review of current concepts. *Transcripts of the 8th Symposium, Care of the professional voice, Part II.* New York: The Voice Foundation.

Wyke, B. (1983). Neuromuscular control systems in voice production. In D. M. Bless & J. H. Abbs (Eds.), *Vocal fold physiology.* San Diego, CA: College-Hill Press.

Wyke, B., & Kirchner, J. A. (1976). *Neurology of the larynx. Scientific foundation of otolaryngology.* London: Heineman Medical Books.

Zay, H. W. (1917). *Practical psychology of voice and life.* New York: Schirmer.

Zemlin, W. R. (1968). *Speech and hearing science.* Englewood Cliffs, NJ: Prentice-Hall.

Zemlin, W. R. (1984, September/October). Notes on the morphology of the human larynx: A tutorial exposition. *The NATS Bulletin, 41*(1).

Zerffi, W. A. C. (1948). Voice reeducation. *Archives of Otolaryngology, 48.*

Zerffi, W. A. C. (1952, September). Methods of finger palpation. *Annals of Otology, Rhinology and Laryngology.*

APPENDIX

■

DISCOVER YOUR VOICE VOCAL EXERCISES

To understand the principles on which these exercises are based, it is necessary to read the chapters relating to them. Making sounds without the concepts behind them would serve no useful purpose.

Feel you can demonstrate each step before moving on to the next. As you warm up your voice, feel everything in place from the very beginning. On days that you are tired or at times when you are getting over a cold, you may need to spend more time with the beginning exercises. I emphasize throughout the book that it is better to do too little than too much.

Several short practice periods are better than working too long at one time. If any exercise is not comfortable or easy, do not fight it. Positive experiences pave the way for what seems difficult at the moment. It is estimated that voices reach their peak of maturation at age 35, older for dramatic voices. Do not try to sound like a 35-year-old when you are 25.

The first five exercises are based on explanations in Chapter I.

Example 1.

"*Huh* — — — — — ——————— —— —''

Example 2.

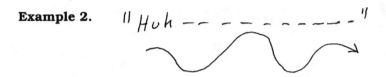

Example 3. Like #2, but continue until out of breath.

Example 4.

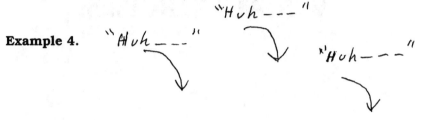

Example 5. Let the sound be as loose and free as a child's laughter.

At this point it is imperative that you read, understand, and practice the exercises for release, posture, and breathing in Chapters II and III. They are the foundation for everything that follows.

In all exercises, try to incorporate the feeling that the tone starts almost before you finish your breath. This helps to maintain a low, firm connection of breath to the tone throughout the exercise.

Between exercises, take a breath for the next scale as you finish the preceding one. In other words, you stop a tone by taking a breath—not stop, empty your lungs and then take a breath. This helps to maintain both chest and larynx in a steady position—no heaving up and down to breathe.

The vowel sounds are represented by the IPA symbols (see Chapter X). A descending sequence of exercises should only carry you as low as is comfortable. Then start over again beginning a bit higher than at first. The sounds should be light, almost breathy at the beginning. An "M" hum (hm) or any freely formed vowel may be used. Let all vowels be pronounced in an easy, childlike manner.

Male voices would start their sounds an octave lower.
See chapter IV for guidelines.

Exercise I

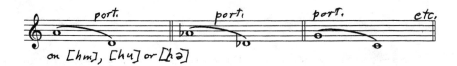

Exercise II

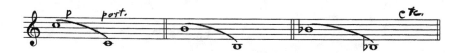

Exercise III

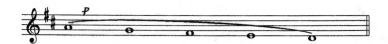

Exercise III a

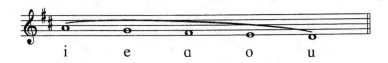

Exercise IV

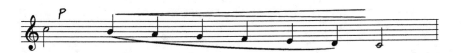

Exercise V

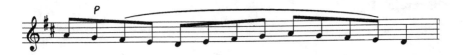

Exercises VI and VII should be done with a steady flow of tone. Try not to jerk from note to note. Let the sixteenth notes float lightly.

Exercise VI

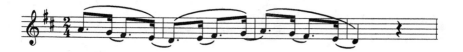

Exercise VII

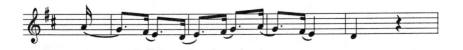

Exercise VIII

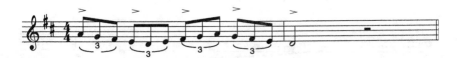

Exercise IX

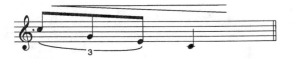

Exercise X

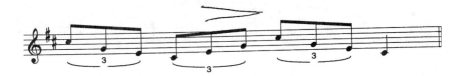

See Chapter V for the following exercises.

To discover the #3 (falsetto) register, start with a light sound at no definite pitch but somewhere above the staff. With the larynx resting low, use a light, breathy sound on either *hoo* (hu), *huh* (hə) or *hum* (hm) and let it slide downwards, like a sigh.

If there is a "break," let the sound be more breathy, softer, and feel the sense of beginning a yawn. This helps the larynx rest in a low position at all times. Refer to the discussion of this problem in the text.

Listen to the audio illustration.

Exercise XI

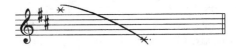

Exercise XII   **Exercise XII a**

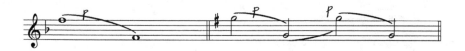

Exercise XIII

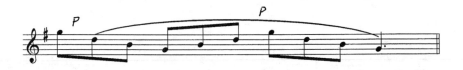

Exercise XIV

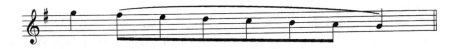

Exercise XIV a

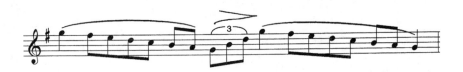

To discover the #1 (vocal fry, pulse) register, let your voice descend in a light, breathy quality. No pushing down! The larynx should rest low and feel very loose.

Exercise XV

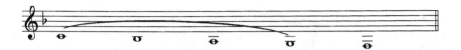

For the #4 (flute, whistle) register, again just think the pitch and let a light flow of air start the sound. The larynx should still rest in a low, relaxed position. No reaching up! With a relaxed jaw, round your lips freely for *oo* (u) and let a flow of air be like cooling your coffee or hot soup.

Exercise XVI

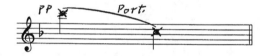

When you have discovered the sound, try exercises XIIa, XIII, and XIV in this range. If the [hu] sound does not work, try a light humming sound, [hm].

Exercises XVII and Exercise XVIIa will help to blend the #2 and #3 registers. This also helps the #4 register as the highest notes are reached.

Notice the light accents on every other note, which avoid an accent on the top note. The top note should be the lightest. Only try the exercise as high as the notes come easily. Your mouth, jaw, and tongue should always be passive. Stretching your mouth open for the top notes or pulling back the corners of your lips will bring tension in your throat. Your larynx will automatically adjust to a thought of pitch if your throat is sufficiently relaxed. The notes should just "pop" out—it will seem to you that you have no control.

Exercise XVII

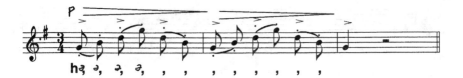

Also try repeating *pup* with a very light sound and loose lips.
[pəpəpəpəp]

Rounding your lips for (u) can help top notes.

Exercise XVII a

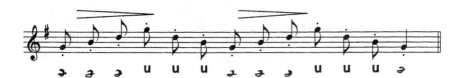

See Chapter VII for the following exercises. I suggest using
the primary Italian vowels in vocalizing: *i, e, a, o, u*. Elicit light,
automatic pitches which adjust to a thought of pitch and a
steady flow of air. Use the vowels that are the easiest. Let the
speed gradually increase until the notes move so fast they seem
out of control. If the pitches are correct, this *is* control because
the notes respond to *thought* and *airflow*, with no muscular set.
Feel a bounce and release from the accented notes.

Exercise XVIII

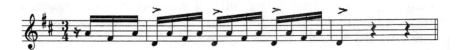

Gradually increase the speed, repeating a number of times as you feel a free bounce.

Exercise XIX

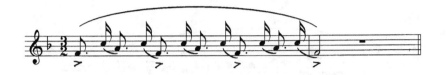

Exercise XIX a

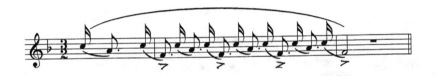

Exercise XX

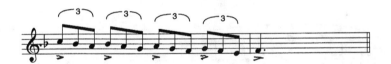

Exercise XX a

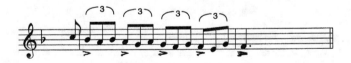

Exercise XX b

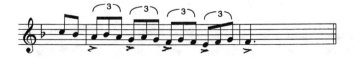

Exercise XXc may be repeated with accents shifted as in XXa and XXb.

Exercise XX c

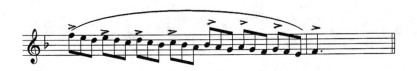

Exercise XXI

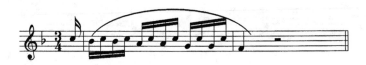

Exercise XXI a

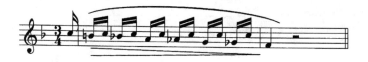

Exercise XXI b

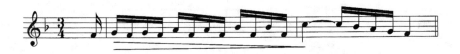

Exercise XXI c

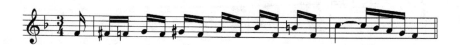

Exercise XXII

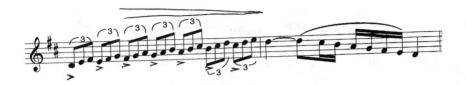

Let the 16th notes in Exercise XXIII be very light.

Exercise XXIII

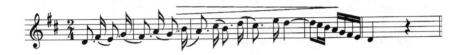

Exercise XXIV

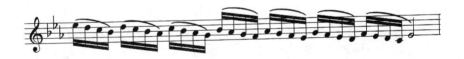

Exercise XXIV a

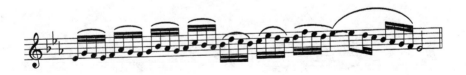

Exercise XXV

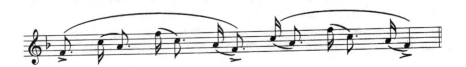

Exercise XXV a

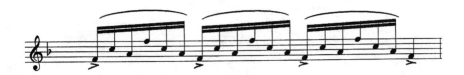

Exercise XXV b

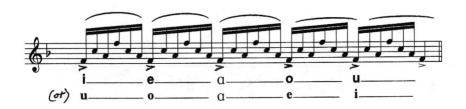

Exercise XXV c

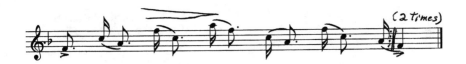

Exercise XXV d

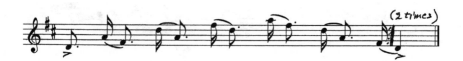

Exercise XXVI is for extending the breath. Only go as far as can be done on *one breath.* Gradually the breath will carry you further as the vocal folds become more efficient in their use of air. Do not expect to carry this through on one breath the first time.

Exercise XXVI

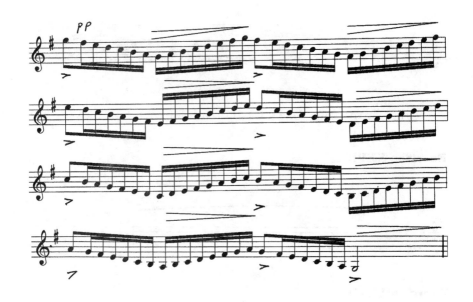

Exercise XXVI a

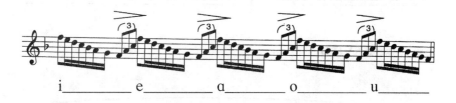

Exercise XXVI b

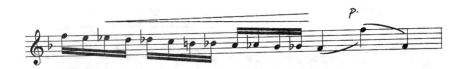

Exercise XXVI c

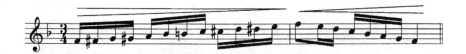

Drills for the trills. Use a fresh breath for each four measures.

Exercise XXVII

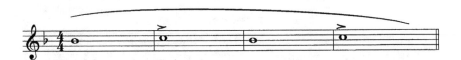

Exercise XXVII a

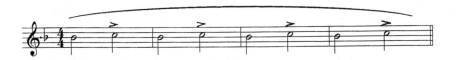

Exercise XXVII b

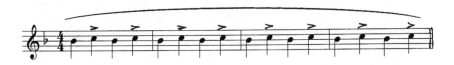

Exercise XXVII c

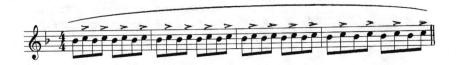

Exercise XXVII d

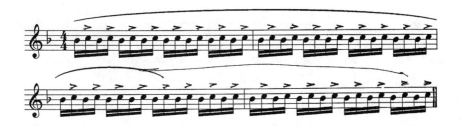

Exercise XXVII e

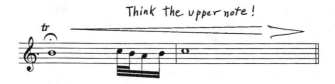

Exercise XXVIII

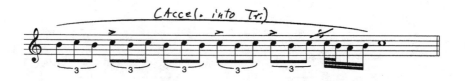

    Starting with Exercise XXVII, the same patterns may be used for the whole note trill.

    Exercise XXIX is also to be done on one breath. In this exercise, avoid crescendo or diminuendo. Exaggerate the legato line, virtually sliding from note to note, like sighing. This exercise is also for blending #3 and #2 registers.

Exercise XXIX

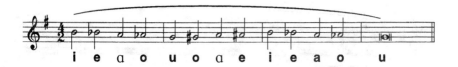

Using the same pattern of vowels, this scale may be expanded by using five whole note intervals; five minor thirds; five major thirds; five perfect fourths.

See Chapter VIII for Exercise XXX.

It will take time to master these new exercises before you can do them on every note in your range. Never let a crescendo grow beyond the point where you can keep a mix of #3 with the #2 register.

These exercises are to be done on one breath.

Standing tall, keep your ribs comfortably expanded, especially toward the end of phrases. Feel a sensation like putting your foot on ice as you start the tone. Let each vowel gradually blend into the next vowel, thus avoiding abrupt changes. Repeat the exercise, moving higher or lower by half steps. (Listen to the audio illustration.)

Exercise XXX

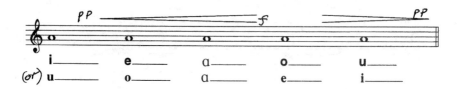

Exercise XXXI

Before you sing the beginning note, in your mind be thinking the pitch of the upper note as you start. Feel that the larynx rests in one position, with the upper note just "popping" out of the same place that the lower one is being produced. Let the upper note be lighter. In time, repeat this rhythmic pattern on wider intervals: a fourth; an augmented fourth; a fifth; a minor sixth; a major sixth, etc.

Exercise XXXI

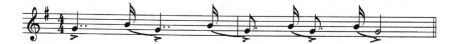

In Exercise XXXII, feel a bounce from the lower note to an unaccented note above. This exercise may also be tried on wider intervals.

Exercise XXXII

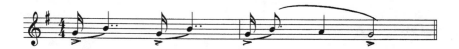

In Exercise XXXIII, feel that the lowest note is the strongest.

Exercise XXXIII

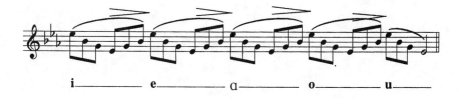

Exercise XXXIV is designed to help form consonants firmly but crisply. A combination of any two consonants with any vowel may be used. For control, try the variation in Exercise XXXIVb, which provides a combination of two sounds in a pattern of triplets musically.

Exercise XXXIV

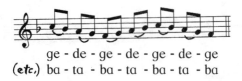

ge - de - ge - de - ge - de - ge
(*etc.*) ba - ta - ba - ta - ba - ta - ba

Exercise XXXIV a

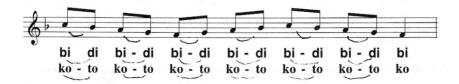

bi di bi - di bi - di bi - di bi - di bi - di bi
ko - to ko - to ko - to ko - to ko - to ko - to ko

Exercise XXXIV b

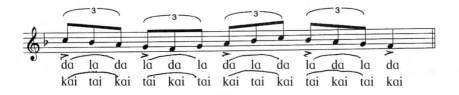

da la da la da la da la da la da la da
kai tai kai tai kai tai kai tai kai tai kai tai kai

INDEX